DEDICATION

For Moira, Carol and Kate.

FIRST CATCH YOUR PATIENT
A Vet on Call

by

R. RUSSELL LYON, BVM&S, MRCVS

PUBLISHED IN GREAT BRITAIN BY
SMALLHOLDER PUBLICATIONS LTD,
HIGH STREET,
STOKE FERRY,
KINGS LYNN,
NORFOLK PE33 9SF

ISBN 1-870573-07-2

Acknowledgements:
Photographs by Anna Oakford
Line Drawings by P. Leicht

Typeset and Printed by
The MANSON Group Ltd
Hemel Hempstead, Herts

CONTENTS

Preface

"MUCH MAY BE MADE OF A SCOTCHMAN, IF HE BE CAUGHT YOUNG."

I cannot remember precisely when I first realised I would like to be a veterinary surgeon. It was a comparatively slow process, complete by the time I was thirteen years old. I got the urge to do something about my ambition, very early one cold winter's morning.

I was born and raised on a mixed arable farm in the Scottish Borders. We had a herd of Ayrshire dairy cows and a flock of breeding ewes, half of which were Blackface and the others were a cross breed known as Greyfaces. That doesn't tell the whole story, as on the farm there were also hens, turkeys, the occasional pig and two ponies in the winter months. The farm was in all, about three hundred acres which varied in parts from a rich loam soil to heather and whin clad moorland.

Our herd of cows were milked twice a day, a process that began just after five o'clock in the morning. It had to start this early as we had to have the milk ready to go away when the lorry came, which was usually about seven thirty in the morning. It would often be quite pleasant to be up and about that early in the summer months, even though this did not quite fit in with my inclination to read half the night.

Winter mornings, cold and dark were, I found, a very different proposition. The morning which crystallised my thoughts and seasoned my ambition was very cold. It was the middle of January. I was carrying a churn full of milk, about four gallons in all, from the warm byre (milking shed) to the milk house where the milk was cooled and then stored in ten gallon cans. The route led along a concrete walkway which at that time in the morning was covered in black ice. I used the same route countless times as there was a lot of milk to carry, but inevitably one of the times I slipped over, fell and the milk went everywhere including over me. As I pulled myself upright my hand stuck to a metal railing, it was so cold.

I was not renowned for my speed of thought even then but in that instant my mind was made up, that I could not and would not do that job for the rest of my working life. I wanted out and as soon as possible.

I had a cousin who was a vet in a large practice near Kelso. As a youngster I spent many of the summer months with him while he was working. He was a quiet, patient man. He needed to be, as he spent much of his time visiting farms and stables. He travelled up to seventy thousand miles a year in pursuit of his patients and he was held in great esteem and affection by all.

My main job when I was with him, apart from fetching and carrying, was to open and close the many farm gates that we encountered. In between calls, we would listen on a very crackly car radio to the "Archers" and the test matches and it is little wonder I am still addicted to both these programmes. It was from him I first got the idea, I would like to be a vet.

I was not thought to be particularly good with animals by my family. My elder brother had a much greater affinity with the beasts on the farm although they all knew to fear him if they stepped out of line. He could literally charm the birds out of the trees or in his case the bantams down from the roof rafters. Our bantams roosted on the wooden beams in the small byre and he could talk to them in their language and they would fly down and perch on his shoulder.

I didn't have the same touch at all. I was given a young sheep dog to train which had shown a lot of promise. In the end, father had to take it away from me and sell it to a cousin who had a large sheep farm before I ruined it completely. He reckoned I was too soft, "kind hearted" were the words he used, to train an animal properly. Although my upbringing gave me a very matter of fact way of dealing with life and death, when I was young, I could never bear to see anything hurt and I'm not much better now.

My passage through the Royal (Dick) School of Veterinary Medicine was not without difficulty and incident. It was largely self financed through summer jobs working as a crop inspector for the Ministry of Agriculture and by my father helping me to carry on farming in a limited way with some sheep and cattle of my own. I never had to pay for their feed and strangely enough none of my animals were ever ill or died. Or if they did, he never told me and made up the numbers from his own animals which was much more likely.

After five years in Edinburgh I qualified, much to my amazement and relief. I was fortunate enough to be offered two jobs in Scotland but I wanted to broaden my horizons a bit and I felt there were better jobs and prospects south of the border. I am fond of quoting Samuel Johnson.

"The noblest prospect which a Scotchman ever sees, is the high road that leads him to England".

In my case this was just about right. I joined a practice in Cambridgeshire. The senior partner was a Scotsman so I felt instantly at home and within a year I was married, a baby was on the way and I had been offered a partnership. It was the start of a career in the Fens where people are as idiosyncratic as they were welcoming. It was a decision I have never regretted and although I miss the hills of home, the Fenland scene has a grandeur all of it's own which after twenty-five years is still, as I found it, stark but beautiful.

[illegible] pay [illegible]

[illegible]

After [illegible] in Edinburgh [illegible] and rather [illegible] in Scotland [illegible]

[illegible] London [illegible]

[illegible]

FIRST - CATCH YOUR PATIENT!

The Fenland Washes that include the vast area between the New and Old Bedford Rivers which run from Earith in Cambridgeshire all the way to the North Sea, are a wildfowler's paradise, a bird watcher's 'heaven on earth' and a fisherman's dream come true. They can also be the scene of a veterinary surgeon's nightmare.

In the summer months, hundreds and perhaps thousands of cattle, horses and sheep are grazed on the rough pasture which in the winter months is often covered with flood water.

An emergency call from one of the shepherds who patrol the grazings, saying that one of their charges is in trouble, often causes a sinking sensation in the vet who has to respond. Mostly when an animal is in trouble the shepherd will have it penned up ready for your visit, but there are occasions when, for a variety of reasons, this just doesn't happen.

It never occurred to me throughout my veterinary training that the first thing I would have to learn when starting rural practice in the Fens, was that there would be times when you would be expected to catch your own patient! Indeed, on my first day in the practice, my boss took me out to the surgery car park, and with the help of a ten gallon oil can as a target, proceeded to show me how it was done! It seems to be a peculiarity of the Fens which can try a vet's patience to the utmost. It was also appears to be a custom that goes back a long way. I have read a diary of a local vet who was practising about one hundred years ago and complained of just the same thing.

It's not that all Fen farmers are mean about buying adequate equipment with which to restrain their beasts, but many just don't see the need for it when a vet can do it perfectly well for them. Indeed, in some farms one is often judged on one's ability with a lasso. Extra points are given for being able to "whirl it" overhead cowboy style, and points deducted if you are actually unsporting enough to wait until the animal stands still. Now all of this can be quite entertaining if your patient is in a closed yard and cannot get too far away from you, but it is quite a different matter when it is in the middle of a large field on Welney Wash!

I can best illustrate the difficulties we veterinary surgeons encounter by recounting an emergency I was called to some time ago. The problem, the shepherd explained when I met him in Welney, was a cow in difficulty having her calf. We drove in his landrover for about three miles down the bank of the Hundred Foot river before he stopped and pointed to a field in the distance with some cows in it. I was handed a pair of binoculars through which I managed to see and assess the difficulties we were facing.

The cow was lying in the corner of a field, straining and trying to give birth, and I could just see two little feet peeping out of the animal's rear end. She had been like that all morning and it was now about mid-day. We discussed our plan of action as to how we were going to catch her. Josh, the shepherd was just a bit pessimistic; "tha'r as wild as hawks master" he said. "I don't know how we are going to get on". The alternative to catching her in the field was to drive the whole herd back up the river bank to the roadside pens. With only two of us to herd them, the possibilities of wild cattle escaping into other fields or even jumping in the river was just too awful to contemplate, so we decided to reconnoitre the scene by vehicle. The cows were used to the landrover moving about them and I hoped they wouldn't take fright. It was humans they ran away from!

We couldn't wait for help to arrive as the problem was an urgent one and needed resolving as soon as possible or the calf would be born dead. Josh took the wheel again and I sat on the large tyre which the vehicle had on its bonnet, with my catching rope at the ready. We approached quietly with the wind behind us as it's easier to throw a rope accurately with the wind in that quarter. All went well at first, we passed through the herd without trouble and got very close to my intended patient where she lay on the ground. She was too pre-occupied with her efforts to expel her burden to take any notice of us. It was at this point I made a cardinal mistake. Just as I threw the lasso she looked round, saw me, and moved her head enough for me to miss her with my first attempt. She got up and moved away suspiciously. We followed her hoping against hope that I would get close enough again to have another shot at getting the rope on her. I should have known better, as it was all to no avail. Our passage around the field after her got faster and faster and more futile by the minute. It was perhaps just as well that I hadn't succeeded with my attempts as I had completely forgotten to consider what I was going to do with the free end of the rope if I had managed to get the noose on her!

We stopped to reconsider our position. In the meantime the patient took herself off to the far corner of the field and resumed grazing as if having a calf was the last thing on her mind. Despair and defeat stared us in the face but the cow and her unborn calf still urgently needed assistance.

Despair I have found however, is often the mother of low animal cunning, and another idea came into my mind. We drove the cow with much shouting and whistling and general uproar, to the edge of the field where it was bounded by a large watercourse full of black mud and water in roughly equal proportions. Into this she jumped as I had hoped, and was instantly stuck fast up to her belly. Now it was easy - I'm quite good with the lasso when the target can't run away!

We soon had her out on dry land with the aid of the landrover to which she was now firmly attached. It was fortunate for all concerned that along with my calving equipment, I also carry a container of clean water and antiseptic. Without wasting any more time, I quickly put some calving ropes on what I discovered to be the front legs of what appeared to be quite a large calf. After making sure that the calf's head was in the correct position and engaged in the pelvis between the front feet, I connected the ropes to the calving machine. This is a T-shaped instrument with the horizontal part placed against the animal hindquarters. The vertical part has a ratchet type of device to which the ropes are attached and then with a lever, tension is applied to the ropes. With this means a consistent pulling action is applied and gradually and carefully the baby was delivered. Great care has to be taken when using this calving jack, as in the wrong hands considerable damage can be caused to both mother and offspring, but the machine is also a great boon as in a situation where there is very little assistance, like this, a calf can be delivered alive that would otherwise have died.

The youngster was soon on his feet, and the cow being a good mother soon took a lively interest in him. She was given a prophylactic injection of penicillin and was let in peace to take charge. Josh reported later in the day that both were doing well.

Usually the animals grazing the Washes spend a trouble free time there, but when a problem occurs it can be very difficult and time consuming to deal with. I was just grateful that for once Mother Nature came to my aid enough to allow me to finish the job to everyone's satisfaction, including the patient's!

You could be forgiven for assuming that it's only in farm animal practice that the vet is going to be faced with the prospect of having to catch the patient. Not so! Many times I have had to crawl under a bed to collect a cat or retrieve a budgie from a curtain top, and one of the strangest cases occurred with a dog.

The day I encountered this particular animal, a shaggy reprobate of a Cocker Spaniel, it was near the end of my morning round. It had been a comparatively quiet morning, which had not been too physical or mind stretching, on a pleasant if dull day for mid-January. I had gone from call to call, accepting the odd cup of coffee here and there (with nothing stronger) and was just contemplating what might be in prospect for lunch, when my cosy complacency was rudely shattered by the crackling squelch of the radio-telephone "Vet Base to Vet One, Vet Base to Vet One" Anne our telephonist, action-desk girl came over the air, with uncharacteristic urgency.

"Vet One to Base, yes Anne, What's the matter?" I asked. I didn't really want to know.

"How soon can you get to Mr Stone's at Whaplode? One of the dogs is trapped in a shaft and they want you to get it out." She replied.

"Which dog is it, Anne?"

"Ben" came the reply, as if it really mattered which one it was. I decided it could have been worse. Not one of my favourite dogs, but it was one of my favourite clients. "Okay Vet Base, tell them I should be there in about fifteen minutes; over and out."

Arriving at the farm I was greeted by farmer Bob and all the Stone family. This in itself showed how seriously they viewed the situation; normally it could take up to twenty minutes to find just one of them! I was conducted round the yard by the distraught owners to the end wall of a new potato store. A hole was pointed out at the base of the wall, which was an opening into a ventilation shaft. It was about a foot square and almost concealed by an elderberry bush which had its roots in a muddy patch. Well, there was nothing else to be done but to get down on all fours in the mud and have a look for myself.

The requested light helped me to see the neurotic animal stuck some three yards along the wooden tunnel. How he came to be stuck facing the exit I couldn't begin to understand. I don't think even Ben would be daft enough to reverse into a hole like that! But well and truly stuck he was, wide-eyed with fear, and whining in exasperation.

I sat on my haunches at the entrance and considered the position. The shaft was too narrow and the dog too far in to be able to get anywhere near it with an arm or any other human appendage with which to pull him out. There was no other way he could come out except the way he went in, unless we moved about five hundred tons of potatoes. The prospect of the manoeuvre didn't exactly thrill me and I was glad to have the idea vetoed by Bob as he said that any movement of the potatoes might dislodge the tunnel and crush the dog.

"Mind you" he said, "how would it be if you injected him with a dart gun, and when he's unconscious I'll send in the terrier with a line attached. Perhaps the line would get tangled up with Ben and then we could pull him out."

"Good thinking" I said, not wishing to be too censorious, "but the only gun I have fires rather lethal lead projectiles." There was a further silence which Bob's wife took for despair on my part.

"Perhaps we should have sent for the Fire Brigade." she said somewhat falteringly. That did it! Spurred on by the thought of defeat and loss of face, the solution when it came to me was simplicity itself. I rushed back to the surgery for the dog catcher, not in this instance one of my fetching quartet of nurses, but the more prosaic metal type; this consists of a tube about five feet long with a rope down the middle and a loop at the end.

Thus equipped, I once more lay in the mud and at arm's length and with the aid of my finger tips, manoeuvred the noose over the bemused dog's head. After a few attempts I had him securely, and with the family's assistance we gave an almighty heave and out he came like the cork out of the proverbial bottle.

Now, that dog and I have never been the best of friends. He always avoided me whenever possible, but I do believe that on this occasion he was actually pleased with what I had done for him; and for the first and probably the last time, he came over to me and totally unbidden, licked my hand. Even so, I do hope that I don't ever have to lie in the mud for him again!

Fire is one of the most frightening natural hazards that animals, and man for that matter have to encounter. Wild animals, when a wood or heathland is on fire, can hope to escape by running in the opposite direction. How much more frightening it must be for domestic animals that are housed in buildings and perhaps tethered. When a fire breaks out they are totally at the mercy of the element unless help is at hand. I have seen some awful sights both during and after fires where, despite valiant efforts by farmer and farm workers many animals have perished. Firemen too have a wonderful record for bravery in trying to rescue stock.

A particular fire I was called to involved a piggery. I arrived when the worst of the blaze was over. Those pigs that had managed to escape were wandering around in a dazed state. All around was the stench of soot and burned flesh, and the general debris of blackened timbers and burned walls criss crossed by fire hoses, and water everywhere.

My attention, however, was drawn to a large drain to one side of the piggery. A group of fireman were gathered at the edge. The drain was steep sided and about six feet down before the water level, and the water itself was the same depth again. I peered over some shoulders to see a large sow swimming serenely up and down the twenty to thirty feet length of the water course, evading all the mens' attempts at catching her with their makeshift lariats made from firehoses.

By now it was semi-dark and a search light from the fire tender followed the animal's progress. She seemed quite unconcerned. Apparently she had been one of the last ones out of the burning building, and had dashed straight over to the water and without hesitation jumped in. A plan was arranged for her capture: I was held securely by the belt of my trousers, by a team of men one behind the other. I balanced precariously over the edge, waiting, lasso at the ready for her to swim by me. I caught her on the third lap and passed the end of the rope back to the team. They very easily and willingly pulled her out, despite her squeals and protests. She was given some treatment for her burns and found accommodation for the rest of the night in what was left of the piggery.

It would be pleasant to report that her efforts had been worthwhile, as it was most eminently sensible of her to seek water for her burns, but I found the next day on my revisit that her injuries were too extensive to treat properly, and she had to be put down on welfare grounds.

Catching your patient is often frustrating, occasionally rewarding, but often as in this last case, has a disappointing outcome.

A HARD DAYS NIGHT

A vet's job is never done, and one of the hard things a new graduate has to come to terms with is the plain fact that after a busy day and sometimes hectic evening, there will be occasions when you will be required to get out of bed on a cold winter's night and attend to a patient. Everyone going into practice realises this, but the reality when it occurs, often comes a great shock to the system. There is little more likely to chill the soul than the telephone ringing in the small hours. It is comparatively easy to answer its summons through the day in an efficient, competent, friendly manner, but it can be another matter when jerked out of a deep sleep or even a pleasant dream.

When I first entered general practice as a young and keen veterinary surgeon, I used to try very hard to be as efficient on the phone through the night as I was in the daytime. This wasn't all that difficult for me as I am a light sleeper and can almost sense when the phone is going to ring. It took some time for me to realise that answering the telephone like this during the night is not such a good idea, as callers got the impression no matter what the time was, there was a vet in the surgery just waiting from their call!

Matters came to head one night when a smallholder client phoned about his sow. I answered the summons with my usual bright manner.

"Veterinary Surgery, can I help you?"

"Yes mate," came the reply "It's Sonny Hill here. I've just had a look at my old Lucy. She's had fifteen lovely piglets but she don't seem quite right. Can you call and look at her in the morning?"

After making sure he didn't want a visit until morning, I gratefully and quickly went back to sleep. It wasn't until the next day that I fully realised that he had wakened me at 3.30 in the morning to give me a routine message. He was genuinely surprised to be told that I wasn't actually in the office all night! From that moment on, my night telephone manner changed and I now sound sleepier than I sometimes feel!

When I first joined the practice, as a large percentage of the clinical work was with pigs, the most common cause of the night calls was due to farmers sitting up with their sows while they were farrowing. At the first hint of trouble they would request assistance, and unlike Mr Hill they would want you in double quick time. One such caller was "Les" from Welney, who sadly now is long dead. He would never use the telephone through the day and would always get a neighbour to make the call if he had a sick pig. However, come late evening, he lost his fear of the instrument. This behaviour may of course have been influenced by the nightly visits he used to pay to his local just down the road! On more than one occasion he had confidently used the village telephone booth and tried to reverse the charges!

Our professional relationship reached its nadir about midnight one night when Les phoned requesting a visit for one of his sows. His pigs were renowned throughout the Fen as the biggest, fattest and worst tempered! He kept them in old railway carriages, which served their purpose reasonably well, and seemed to be scattered at random about his muddy yard. On his return home from the pub he had checked his animals as per usual before turning in for the night, only to discover one he thought was dying. The reason for this diagnosis according to Les, was that normally when he looked at this particular animal she would bark and chase him out of the shed. This time she lay in her bed, and unlike me wouldn't be roused! Against my better judgement I got out of bed and travelled the twelve miles to his farm. I found Les anxiously waiting in the yard, and together we went in to inspect the dying pig. Sure enough there she was, flat out, oblivious to the world. I climbed in beside her and commenced my clinical examination by taking her temperature: I inserted the thermometer into her rectum, where upon she woke up with a start, and true to form ferociously chased us both for our lives. She had only been asleep all the time! I had always thought Les fed his sows to exhaustion, and here was the proof. Fortunately she was too fat to catch us, but it was a close call. After this episode, whenever Les called at night, my first thoughts tended to be how best to help him without actually getting out of bed!

These days, with the pig industry sadly depleted in this area, the most likely source of a night call is one from the police. These are usually because of a traffic accident to a dog or cat, but the exceptions are always fairly memorable.

A police summons is usually routine and matter of fact, with the call for assistance coming through a central control system. This relays a message and requires only an assurance that I will attend, with an approximate time of arrival at the scene.

One night the nuance of the message was slightly bemusing. A mildly amused controller asked me to attend a road traffic accident to a "small furry animal." I was intrigued even though it was 1.30am, and sufficiently awake to take a fishing net and a pair of gloves with me. I didn't have to travel far, only about two hundred yards from my own door, to discover two policemen looking decidedly uncomfortable, standing guard over a car which had ran into a tree on a perfectly straight piece of road. The driver claimed he had not been drinking but had swerved to avoid a little cream coloured creature which had ran across the road.

"We have to believe him, because there it is now under that bush," one of the policemen said.

By peering into the undergrowth with the help of a powerful torch, I could just make out a pair of small bright orange eyes gazing up at me. Investigating further, I discovered a fully grown male Polecat Ferret totally unconcerned about the havoc he had wreaked on the highway, but quite happy to be picked up and deposited in the cat basket I had brought along for the purpose. He was totally unscathed, and very friendly, much to the relief of the attending constables, who had been wondering whether to tie up the bottoms of their trouser legs just in case of trouble!

Felix the Ferret was put in the surgery and happily lived there for two or three days on cat food, until I had worked out who the owner might be and arranged for his safe return. I'm still not sure how the insurance claim for the car worked out!

Not many road traffic accidents end as happily as that one, particularly those that happen at night. One recent case which caused a lot of heartache was the result of horses getting out of what was thought to be a secure field. No one can explain to this day how the gate came to be open, but foul play by person or persons unknown is suspected. The owners of the horses were abroad at the time but had left a very responsible locum tenens in charge who had fed and cared for them. This particular dark wet night, both horses got out of the open gate. They galloped about half a mile to a main road where, with all the predictability of Sod's Law, they ran full tilt into a passing car. The car driver, understandably shocked, said that he saw neither animal until they loomed out of the dark and collision was inevitable and unavoidable. One horse was killed virtually outright and was certainly dead when I arrived on the scene. The other had an awful gaping chest wound. The car driver had to be carted off to hospital, and the car was a total write-off.

Fortunately, the injured horse eventually made a good recovery, but the sight of that dead animal lying in a pool of blood on the black wet road with the rain pouring down, will remain with me for a long time. At least the car driver survived, it could so easily have been him who was killed. Perhaps the accident could have been totally avoided if the gate had been padlocked as well as bolted; but then it's always easy to be wise after the event.

Night calls for horses are not uncommon, especially around foaling time and I have on many occasions been called to assist in the delivery of a foal. When all is well, and mother is delivered of a healthy offspring it's always an occasion for some celebration, even if it's only a cup of coffee from a grateful client. Most owners, if the mare has managed to have the foal by itself, will leave ‘phoning for the antenatal check up until morning. One night was different.

A lady whom I knew to be a non panicking, sensible owner phoned just after I had gone to bed. The tone of her voice told me that something was terribly wrong. She informed me that the mare had foaled and asked me to come straight away. I didn’t question her; I tumbled out of bed and broke all the speed limits to get to her stables just as quickly as possible, The mare had indeed given birth to a healthy colt foal. Its hind feet were still inside the mare’s body. The mare herself was quite dead from a massive internal haemorrhage. She was still warm, her muscles were still twitching with the final heroic effort she had given while dying, to ensure her foal would live. But she was beyond any recall.

We got the foal on his feet and dried him off. He nuzzled his dead mother, obviously hungry. I milked the colostrum out of the mare’s udder and because we had no feeding bottle or teat to hand, we used the time honoured method of using a rubber glove and cut the end off a finger to use as a teat. This served him well and kept him going until morning when we managed to get some artificial mares milk. He was hand reared into a strapping and lively animal who now looks marvellous, and cheeky with it, and belies his hazardous journey into life. I can never look at him, however, without recalling his mother, who died while giving him life.

One of the most bizarre night calls I have ever had happened last year, at the height of the hot weather. A couple, who like most of us when it’s hot at night, were asleep with their bedroom window wide open, when their cat came into the room. The husband woke up, hearing a slight kerfuffle and scratching noises, to see that the cat had brought another visitor as well. It was, would you believe, a rat! Not only that, having brought the rodent into the house, Puss decided that his night’s work was done, and went to sleep in his basket. By this time, the wife, now awake, shot up in bed and screamed quite loud enough to waken the neighbourhood, as well as the family dog who just happened to be asleep in the bedroom at the time. The dog, smartly perceiving the cause of the uproar, promptly grabbled the rat and killed it.

“Wonderful,” thought the husband, “what a good dog.” He gingerly got out of bed, seized the rat by the tail and slung it out of the open window; only for it to be closely pursued by the dog! The lady of the house screamed again. The bedroom was on the first floor and all they heard was the thump of the dog hitting the driveway, and then silence. The husband, aghast at his folly, couldn’t bring himself to go downstairs and look at his dog, he obviously feared the worst.

Eventually he called me, then went downstairs and opened the front door to be greeted by the dog sitting on the door step, wagging his tail! On closer inspection he was none the worse for his "flight" and was only stiff for a day or two afterwards as the result of bruising.

The most difficult, arduous night I ever spent in the pursuit of my calling happened when I wasn't even on duty! A colleague phoned me about one in the morning with a daft question.

"Are you doing anything much at the moment?" I very nearly said I was but hastily reconsidered, because if I was I wouldn't be telling him anyway! He was calling from the mobile phone we carry on such occasions, from Welney Wash, and had been there since 9.30pm trying to calf a heifer cow. The calf was dead inside the beast and he, the vet, was totally exhausted from trying to get it out. I obtained directions from him, which didn't sound too promising! I had to drive down a cart track for about two miles and then walk a further three hundred yards to the field where they were. I would see his car and the farmer's truck and torches in the distance when I was getting close.

It was very dark, wet and windy night, and I remember cursing the farmer for his folly of having a heifer which was due to give birth in such a difficult and out of the way location. When I arrived at the field the animal was tied to a fence in what was now a muddy corner, and she looked as exhausted and miserable as everyone else. Not that I could see too much, as the light from the torches were beginning to fade somewhat. There was at least plenty of assistance; three others were there to help, which included the farmer, as well as my colleague. I had taken some water with me to augment what they already had and with that I scrubbed up, having reluctantly removed my jacket and donned the obstetrical gown, and set to work.

It was very evident that I would have to do an embryotomy on the calf. This means, in simple terms, cutting up the dead calf whilst it is till in the mother' womb, before removing it in bits.

This procedure is used quite frequently when a foetus is dead and it cannot, for any one of a multitude of reasons, be assisted from the uterus in the normal way. It saves the mother the trauma of a caesarean operation. It's a long, difficult, strenuous job at the best of times, made worse that night by the awful weather. As I worked, I reflected on the fact that the only warm part of me was my arms, which were most of the time, plunged inside the poor cow! How well she earned that unfortunate description.

With every groan from the beast, the owner, who was by this time in great despair and distress for his animal, would disappear into the darkness, and we seriously considered at one point whether he was preparing to throw himself in the river, which was just over the bank from where we were working! I knew he was squeamish, as he once before at another calving (in his yard at home this time), fainted at a vital moment! On that occasion he was holding the halter that was tethering the cow to a post: I delivered the calf after some difficulty. It was alive, I turned to tell Jack of his good fortune, but he was flat out! Oblivious to everything, but to give him his due, he still had hold of the rope while he lay on the ground!

This night seemed to be without end for everyone, and it must have seemed an eternity to the cow. To make matters worse, I had to decide that she would have to go for slaughter in the morning, as she had sustained internal damage which would make it uneconomical for her to be retained within the herd. Such are the hard, unsentimental decisions that vets and farmers have to make from time to time about the animals in their care. That night made such an impact on my veterinary colleague, that he not long afterwards left the practice for the comfort and comparative quietness of a small animal practice.

There are a few times when a night time call does not necessitate a visit. The last time this happened, I remember looking at my watch, it was 4am. I had great difficulty in hearing what the caller had to say, as there was an almighty storm raging outside. I managed to understand that the gale's campaign of fury had met with some success, and had blown off a piggery roof. The fattening pigs within were in some distress, and were finding it difficult to shelter from the elements. Miscellaneous bits of building were still being blown about. In short, they were turning blue with cold, and shivering violently. Could I help? My only rational thought, and I admit it took me a few minutes to think of it, was for the farmer to throw as much straw as possible into the building among the animals. This would, I reasoned, give them as much protection as possible given the circumstances. The suggestion was greeted with a snort of derision and the comment that he had already tried that! The straw had blown out of the shattered building as fast as it could be thrown in. A further few minutes were spent discussing the problem, and then I came to the conclusion that as far as could be determined, the pigs in the building were uninjured and there wasn't much anyone could do until dawn, or until the storm abated. To this conclusion my caller agreed, and confessed that he had known this really when he called me, but he needed someone to talk to and he knew I wouldn't mind being disturbed! He was right, for once, I didn't mind at all, but I did feel more than a little guilty about snuggling back into a warm bed when I knew that not very far away, a large number of pigs were having a very miserable night.

PIGS MIGHT FLY

When I first came upon this Fenland scene as a fully fledged veterinary surgeon, I was about as useful to the practice that I had joined as a boil on the back of the neck. I was made aware at the outset that I had become a member of, what was probably at that time, the largest pig practice in the country. This wasn't our estimate, but that of the local Ministry of Agriculture, from whom we obtained supplies of Crystal Violet vaccine. This vaccine was used before a slaughter policy was instituted, to control Swine Fever Disease.

The fact that the practice was principally in the business of treating pigs didn't worry me too much, as being young and keen, I overlooked the fact that I hardly knew one end of a pig from the other! I was soon to learn — and lanced the boil.

A great number of pigs were kept by farmers and smallholders, but more than a few were in huts (rarely grand enough to be called sties) at the bottom of the garden. This had many advantages for the owners, as they were a ready source of food when slaughter time came around, as well as being useful repositories for the family scraps from the table. This latter habit is now illegal if the waste food contains meat products. Any scraps that are not of vegetable only origin, should be boiled for a specified length of time before being

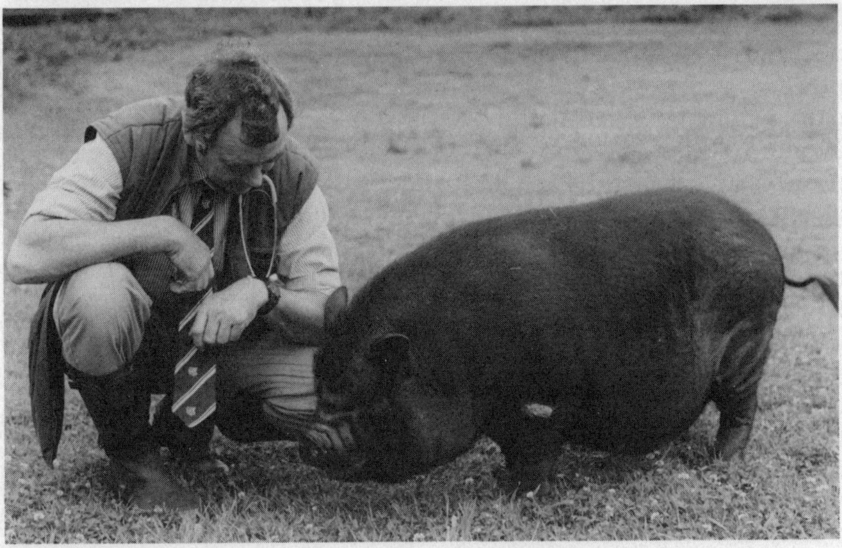

Anna Oakford

The Author chats to "Berkeley" the Vietnamese Pot Bellied Pig.

fed, according to Ministry regulations. Needless to say this didn't always happen, and as a consequence pigs would become infected with Foot and Mouth disease or Swine Fever, as the virus of these diseases often lie dormant in meat products, especially if the meat originated from abroad. Both diseases could be widely spread and cause havoc to the pig population before diagnosis, but be controlled by vaccination or slaughter of infected stock, and very strict movement restrictions.

It was not uncommon, having fed a pig at the bottom of the garden, that when it came to killing time and having made a pet of the animal, the family couldn't bear to give the order and the animal would live on for years, getting larger and larger. Such was the case in a council house garden to which I was called to attend a sow. She was in terminal heart failure due to age and obesity. Within 24 hours she died, and the question was raised, "How do we dispose of the body?" On a farm the answer used to be simple. You called a knacker man and he would happily oblige and remove the carcass. In this case the only way in or out of the back garden was through the front door into the hallway, through the kitchen and out of the back door! To drag a large, dead pig up the garden, through the house and into the street before loading it into a van was clearly not on! I had to give the order for it to be buried in the garden, and it took the man of the house assisted by sundry (or was it surly) children, two days to dig a hole deep enough and complete the job. Needless to say they never felt the need to rear another pig and the sty reverted to being a potting shed.

Most people who owned a few pigs in those days, always felt it necessary to sit up with them when they were giving birth. It's a habit nowadays almost completely done away with, as pig farmers employing labour can't afford to pay for someone to sit up all night! Modern technology has also made it unnecessary, as it is now possible to inject the expectant mother with hormones so that she gives birth during the day, which is much more convenient all round.

Being on night duty 20 years ago meant that if the phone rang in the night, the chances were it would be because of a sow or gilt having problems farrowing. Occasionally, the difficulty was not in having the piglets, but because the sow was savaging them. Some sows seemed to be able to consume their offspring just as fast as they could produce them! I often used to wonder if her deranged behaviour was not due at least in part to the unnatural surroundings in which she was being forced to give birth, while being watched into the bargain.

The answer to combat this enraged behaviour of the sow was to rush along and anaesthetise the mother until she had finished farrowing. Most of the time, when she woke up, she had forgotten what she was so angry about and got on with the job of feeding her family. Not every farmer deemed it necessary to call in the vet to a nasty sow. Many used the tried and tested method of feeding two to four pints of beer or Guinness. Happy was the pigman who lived near the pub that would give him the slops for this, obviating the need for him to buy good beer to do the same job.

Another ingenious method of preventing savaging that I recall, was invented by a Lithuanian pig farmer called Gustav who reared pigs just few minutes from the surgery. He devised a halter like system that fitted around the animal's head, which incorporated within its structure a bolt like piece of metal. When the sow opened her mouth to bite the piglet, the bolt would dig into her head just behind her ear. This in theory, made the sow change her ways, but I was never totally convinced by the efficacy of the system. Fortunately, or not, depending on how you look at things, the contraption never gained favour in the rest of the Fens, despite Gustav's fervent advocacy. Gustav finally, disillusioned with pigs, went to Australia taking his system with him.

It should be remembered when handling any domestic animal, and some pigs in particular, that they all have their breaking points, and push them beyond it, their veneer of domesticity will fall from them and they will became like their ancestors, raving dangerous beasts! You should never go into an adult pig's pen, housing a sow or boar, without having some means of defence or retreat. A boar in particular can, with its tushes set at an easy angle for the job, rip you apart. And I mean this quite literally. The rule of self protection is easy to state, and just as easy to forget, as I know only too well! The first time I broke the rule, I nearly paid for it dearly. I had been treating a sow for Erysipelas; this is a disease which causes the animal to have a high temperature, and generally feel very unwell. When I saw her on day one, she was out for the count. Her temperature was 106F, and she had typical diamond shaped, raised skin blotches. I treated her with a jab of penicillin and she didn't as much as blink an eye. On day two I went back, and unable to find the owner, went to find the patient for myself. She was where I had left her the previous day, still apparently asleep. I took her temperature and noted with approval that it was now down to normal; and still she slept on. I decided to give her another injection, and having filled the syringe, thrust the needle into her rear end. That was as far as I got. She leapt to her feet, screaming with outrage, and came for me with a wicked gleam in her eye and malicious intent. I thrust my pig bag containing all my equipment into her open mouth and leapt for safety over the wall before she had time to spit it out. I shook for days after that, and it taught me a lesson I haven't forgotten!

Farrowing time is probably the most stressful time for the pigkeeper, and the animals under his care. But whether a unit becomes and remains viable, depends much more on the other end of the cycle — procreation. It used to be sufficient to allow the weaned sows to run with the boar and let nature take its natural course. Nowadays this is rarely allowed to happen. Boar and sows are separated except for the act of mating although they are allowed to frustrate each other first by keeping within sight, and more importantly smell of one another. The pigman first checks that the sow is fully in season and ready for the boar, by pressing on her back with both hands, or in some cases by sitting on her back. If she gives every indication of liking this activity, by standing with all four feet firmly anchored to the ground, she is deemed to be ready. Boar and sow will then be allowed to meet, where a little foreplay is allowed, fully supervised, of course. Usually, the boar will make all the running with teeth chomping and much salivating, interspersed with the occasional playful nudge in the ribs. This last can be harmful if he hasn't had his toshes (teeth) attended to. When the foreplay gives way to the full act, it is even more essential that they are still watched carefully. It is not uncommon for a boar to be mounted and giving every appearance of satisfaction, when his energies are being directed into quite the wrong orifice, and this doesn't do a lot for conception rates! Normally, what comes naturally is problem free, but if you haven't been careful about selecting the right mate for the sow, serious trouble can ensue. If you put a young inexperienced boar to an old sow, and he shows his inexperience by being clumsy or slow, she is quite likely to turn on him, give him a good hiding, and put him off sex for life! Equally, an old heavy boar can badly hurt a young, small gilt by over robust behaviour.

It is quite common practice now to avoid these difficulties and do away with the boar altogether, and fertilise the sows by artificial insemination. The same principles are applied to check whether the sow is in season, and this is often augmented with a burst of boar odour from an aerosol can. A rubber catheter is used which closely resembles a boar's penis. It is one of those objects in which reality is stranger than fiction, as a boar's penis at its furthest extremity resembles a corkscrew. When a sow is fully in season and receptive, this spiral shaped arrangement, if you will pardon the expression, screws into the cervix and locks in position. When A.I. first came in, I spent quite a bit of time demonstrating the technique to local farmers. One man in particular was very anxious to learn the method, but was somewhat impatient. Once the canula is in position, the bottle containing the semen is attached and the liquid allowed to drain by gravity into the sow. This process can take up to thirty minutes to accomplish. I demonstrated this with the first sow, but when it came to his turn to try he couldn't resist squeezing the bottle to hurry the process along. By doing this, half the quantity of semen was ejected from the sow. I, of course, put him right, told him the error of his ways and said he would be lucky to get any piglets from this sow, or at best a very reduced litter number. I made the mistake at this point of recording which sow I had done, and which was his. In due time when the piglets arrived, my sow had six pigs and his fifteen, and thereafter he stuck to his own technique. So much for the expert!

Over the years, I have worried about the way we look after our domestic animals, and pigs in particular. As pig prices get worse in real terms year by year, farmers have been driven to reduce costs wherever possible. This has resulted in sows for example, no longer being kept in large strawed yards, but instead confined in stalls, usually tethered throughout their pregnancy, only able to stand up or lie down, but not turn around. They are fed once a day. When the system is working properly, the sows look well, but many of the animals are like zombies and some develop manic behaviour patterns, playing endlessly with water drinkers and chewing the metal bars of the cubicle. New legislation has banned the building of any more of these systems and existing stalls are to be phased out by the end of the 1990's. What we must try to ensure is that any new methods devised for the keeping of sows, doesn't recreate some of the worst aspects of the older ways, or create new unsuspected means of distressing the animals under our care. Sows kept in farrowing crates for the short time of giving birth, and for a week or two afterwards, I don't mind nearly so much. The sow can't injure her piglets so easily (intentionally or otherwise) and the stockman can carry out routine tasks in safety to benefit all concerned. However, these crates should have at least some straw provided, as one of the saddest things is to see a sow trying to make a nest in a farrowing crate, where the surface is bare concrete, or at best rubber matting.

Deprived of even the smallest amount of bedding, she will rub her nose raw before she has to give up and produce her litter. Most pigs that are reared for bacon and pork, at some time in their lives are treated for disease with antibiotics. Many pigs fattened indoors, due to bad housing conditions, require antibiotics in their feed as a routine prevention measure, in order to control diarrhoea or pneumonia. These drugs must be stopped before the given slaughter date in order that any residues are clear from their systems before killing. It is often a race against time, hoping they will make it to the end of the withdrawal date and slaughter before pneumonia hits them again.

Recently, the welfare lobby and economic factors have caused farmers to look again at pigs being kept and reared outdoors in very simple shelters. When done correctly it seems to work very well, and diseases like pneumonia and scours are very much reduced, compared to their cousins kept indoors. It's also very delightful to see how pigs enjoy themselves kept in a more natural environment where they are free to socialize, root in the earth and be omnivorous again. They also have their young in the privacy of their own farrowing arks, and have very little trouble indeed. Youngsters born in this open way have a wonderful early life (providing care is taken against natural predators like foxes). To see them play in the open air is as much fun for the spectator as it is for the piglet!

One modern trend which I find appalling is the fashion which has come to us from the Unites States, of keeping miniature pigs as house pets. These are usually Vietnamese Pot Bellied pigs and as they are intelligent, they can usually be toilet trained and will go for walks. But a pig is a pig and should never be used as a "smart" substitute for a dog.

I have a client, who until recently, had a Pot Bellied pig which he had from a very young age. He kept her both indoors and outdoors and made a great fuss of her, even picking her up and cuddling her, until she became too fat to lift! When she was about three years old, she suddenly turned against him, and would bite and chase him whenever the opportunity arose. He had to don cricket pads and brandish a long brush to keep her away from him when he went into her paddock! Matters came to a head one day after a particularly vicious attack. He was so frightened of her, he 'phoned and asked me to put her down. Fortunately, I managed instead, to find a new home for her, and she now lives quite happily in a grass field with a hut for shelter and another Vietnamese reject for company.

I suppose it's asking too much of human nature to expect that all animals will always be kept in a fitting manner. The need to make a profit from them sometimes gets in the way of good husbandry. I am encouraged, however, by the increasing interest in welfare, the expansion of outdoor pig production, and to think that pigs might not really "have to fly" in the future and a vast majority will be kept in a decent, sympathetic environment, and in a manner which they deserve.

AND SHEEP MAY SAFELY GRAZE

Sheep farming over recent years has suffered few of the tribulations to affect the pig industry. Due to Government subsidies, sheep breeding and rearing has been quite profitable and certainly rewarding. Improvements in management have largely been due to better breeding and feeding systems coupled with a trend to indoor lambing. The latter can be a great boon to both the shepherd and his flock, as there is little more miserable than lambing outdoors when the weather is bad. Mutton and lamb is still the most likely meat to be produced by organic methods; growth promoters and antibiotics are not widely used. I do hope in the future the farmers will continue rearing "natural" lamb, as sheep do not take easily to intensive farming.

The annual cycle in ovine agriculture, for me, starts in the Autumn when the ewe comes into season. This triggering of the oestrous cycle is begun by the decreasing amount of daylight affecting sensory areas of the brain. Sheep generally speaking are very fertile creatures, and a ram or tup (the name for the male of the species depending on which part of the country you come from) put to them at this time, providing he is fertile, will mean lambs being born in the spring of the next year. This is some 147 days or about five months after conception.

Rams are remarkable creatures. They behave in the most innocuous way throughout the year, but when it comes to tupping time their powers of fertility and libido are truly amazing! It has been known for a ram to successfully impregnate up to 30 ewes in a day. This sort of achievement can be easily verified as most shepherds fit a harness with marking fluid or a crayon around the tup. This is called a "raddle" and when the ewe is served the evidence of the occurrence is there for all to see, marked on the base of the tail. This is essential knowledge for the farmer as he will then know when that group of sheep will be due to lamb. The colour will be changed regularly, so that very soon over the field where mating is taking place, there will be groups of sheep with different coloured bottoms. No privacy here!

Most commercial ewes will produce twin lambs and often triplets, and this is what farmers in lowland areas are happy to see. In hill country where the living isn't so easy for the sheep, a single lamb is preferred. Attempts have been made at research establishments to produce sheep that will have up to five lambs at a time. One particular breed, the Finnish Landrace will manage this. They have never caught on commercially as the lambs are weak and need a lot of care. In recent times a lot of effort has gone into inducing ewes to come into season earlier so that they lamb around Christmas and the New Year. Their offspring are ready for the table around Easter, which usually ensures the farmer a better price. A simple method of doing this is do introduce a vasectomized ram into the flock during September. These animals are known as teasers for obvious reasons! Their presence stimulates the ewes into an earlier season which they usually all have at about the same time, thus shortening the eventual lambing period. One particular ram I performed this operation on turned out to be a magnificent animal with the finest set of horns you could hope to see on a sheep. He was called "Big Business" and he lorded it over his flock every year with significant pride. I'm sure he would have been mortified to know he could only fire blanks! This teaser system is partially successful, and cheap. A vasectomized ram will live and work for years, but their use will only enable ewes to lamb in late February or early March, and it is better if you want lambs to be born earlier than this to use hormone treatment. With this method, hormone impregnated sponges are inserted into the ewes' vagina up to six weeks before normal breeding time. These are left in situ for fourteen days and in addition a hormone derived from pregnant mares is injected on day twelve. The sheep then have a normal oestrous (season) when the sponges are removed. If they are then served by a fertile ram, and if the shepherd has got his dates worked out correctly, the first lambs will be born around Christmas. Having successfully got the ewe pregnant, the farmer's whole endeavour is to make sure she arrives in the lambing shed or field well, and still pregnant.

There are many hazards along the way which make this journey in time very dangerous for the sheep. During the Summer and Autumn, a particular pest is the blowfly. These insects lay their eggs in soiled and wet wool, usually around the sheep's hind quarters. It is bad husbandry to allow sheep to have dirty bottoms as these regions become very attractive to the fly. The eggs hatch out into maggots and can, if undetected, eat the sheep alive in two to three days. A shepherd must be alert at all times to this possibility, but especially when the weather is wet and humid. Affected animals will be apart from the others, not eating and generally looking miserable. Sheep are routinely dipped, which means totally immersed in a bath of insecticide to try and prevent, amongst other things, blowfly damage. This is effective for only a relatively short time, and at the first hint of trouble this dipping may have to be repeated whether the animal is pregnant or not. However, new "pour on" or spray preparations have reduced the need to dip.

Some years ago I had to attend several sheep who were badly affected by fly strike. As a result of neglect, several sheep were found dead, having been eaten alive by maggots, and others had been so severely damaged they had to be put down. What was certain was that they had all suffered appallingly. The shepherd who was supposed to be looking after the flock was successfully prosecuted for allowing his charges to suffer as they did, and he was fined a considerable sum of money. Strangely enough, he was not banned from looking after livestock, and farmers still continued to employ him. I'm not sure whether they did so because they couldn't get anyone else, or perhaps the collective thought was that as he had been caught once he would be more careful in the future!

Sheep at any time are vulnerable to marauding dogs. A dog need not be large or fierce to do a lot of damage. A small yappy terrier can just as easily stampede a flock and do untold harm, due to stress induced abortions. Nevertheless, the most extreme danger is from packs (two or more) of larger dogs, who may start out chasing a flock just for fun, but very soon the situation can deteriorate into mayhem where individual sheep are cornered, and are caught and mauled. In the worst instance sheep will die with their throats torn out or are so badly injured that the only humane measure is to put them down. It is little wonder given these circumstances, that farmers are allowed in law to shoot any dog found in a field of sheep unattended.

A few years ago, I was out walking in the Scottish Border hills, about 20 miles from any civilisation and enjoying the solitude with my little Border Terrier bitch. I was overtaken on a hill path by a shepherd on a three wheeler bike with a gun strapped to the back of the machine. He stopped and greeted me courteously and said that I had just made his day. Had my dog not been on the leash he was under orders to shoot her as they had been greatly troubled by dogs worrying ewes and killing lambs. Apparently it is quite common for hill walkers to walk with their dogs off the leash, and two had run off in the last few weeks and caused a lot of trouble. I didn't tell him that if he had tried to shoot my dog he would have to have shot me first, but his message certainly made an impact! I do wish more people who walk in the countryside would be more aware of the potential risks, and even if their pet is completely reliable and quiet, always keep it on the lead where there is any possibility of livestock being about.

Sheep worrying by dogs is another good reason for attempting to have a National Registration Scheme for all dogs and not only Pit Bull Terriers, Rottweillers and the like. There are many occasions when dogs who are caught in the act of chasing and killing sheep, are shot and more often than not there is no means of identifying them or their owners. If registration was compulsory for all dogs, then the owner could be traced and held accountable for their animals' behaviour. Some heavy fines, well publicised, would do much to reduce the "pool" of stray and latch key dogs from which the majority of sheep worrying pests are drawn.

Sheep as a species are hardy creatures, but they do make poor patients and have an alarming tendency at times to die mysteriously with nothing but a little froth on their lips to explain their demise. These deaths are often due to infection by clostridical bacteria, which is difficult to demonstrate at post mortem. These particular germs have many different sub types and cause tetanus, botulism and gangrene in people. In sheep there are up to nine different diseases that are known to be the result of clostridical bacteria infections. Some of the diseases have quite picturesque and often self explanatory names such as Pulpy Kidney disease. Clostridium Perfringens type D bacterial toxin, which is the poison secreted from the germ, attacks the kidney and causes it to go soft and pulpy. The sheep then dies of kidney failure and toxaemic shock.

Braxy is a disease caused by Clostridium Speticum and can have a very high mortality. At post mortem very little can be found except perhaps some reddening of the stomach wall. In days gone by such animals when found dead would be eaten by the farmer or shepherd and his family, without apparent ill effect, but it's not a practice I would care to recommend or follow.

The list of diseases goes on, with Black Disease, Blackleg, Dysentery and so on, with many local variations. The point of mentioning all the foregoing is that all these diseases can be so easily prevented by vaccination. A cure when the illness has struck is still virtually impossible. The vaccine is still relatively cheap and easily administered and most farmers will be sensible and make full use of it. There are some, however, who for reasons of economy or forgetfulness don't use it and their livestock can pay a terrible price.

It doesn't matter which stage of pregnancy the ewes may be at, there is always a pest lurking somewhere to take advantage of their vulnerability. Enzootic abortion caused by a Chlamydia Bacteria has been a source of bother, I suspect from when sheep were first herded together. What makes this infection particularly nasty is the risk that this organism can pose to women of a child bearing age. Ewes aborting as the result of this infection get over the illness relatively quickly and painlessly. This is not so for women; shepherdesses, farmers' wives and female vets are all potentially at risk, and can be severely ill following infection as a result of contact with pregnant sheep. Like the clostridial diseases, a good vaccine is available against this abortive agent, but even vaccinated and otherwise healthy animals could be potential carriers of the infection. Current public health advice to all pregnant women is to avoid contact, direct or indirect with any ewes that are in lamb.

It is increasingly common nowadays for sheep to give birth, if not indoors, at least in large enclosed yards. This has proved a great blessing to man and beast alike, as no one can tell me there is an intrinsic value in freezing on a hillside or fenland field while giving birth or attending. However, this modern practice does have its hazards, not the least due to a condition called Pregnancy Toxaemia. This is a metabolic disease which is the result of bad management and an incorrect feeding system. Ewes can become severely ill in the latter stages of pregnancy due to an increased demand for energy. If you feed a sheep too well too early in pregnancy, it will become too fat and by the time it needs extra energy from its diet in late pregnancy, it may not be available, or it may not be able to eat enough for its requirements. Its body attempts to make up for the deficit by converting the body fat into energy; this unfortunately does not work as the fat is converted instead into ketone which poisons the sheep's metabolic system. The answer to the problem is to start the sheep on a low level of nutrition and build it up slowly during the pregnancy so that you are feeding adequate amounts which the ewe can eat and digest in the last few weeks. Exercise too is all important.

Some two to three years ago a client decided after years of lambing outdoors to house all her in-lamb ewes in the run up to lambing. She bought them all in from a freezing cold field and housed them in a cosy straw filled yard; and it was a disaster! Within a few days she had a big problem with sheep becoming severely ill with Pregnancy Toxaemia, as the energy demands had completely changed. The very sick animals were difficult to treat. Oral drenches of glucose solutions were the order of the day - and night, and the worst affected had to be given intravenous drips. Despite this intensive and desperate therapy two of the sheep died and three others had to be aborted early in order to save their lives. All the others in the group, the mildly affected and even the healthy ones were made to go out for a walk twice a day as the exercise seemed to have a real value in preventing any more going down with the disease. Needless to say the animals themselves were quite disgusted by the whole idea and couldn't see the point of it at all, and I'm not sure the farmer was totally convinced either, but I am sure it saved lives. I was reminded at the time of an old fashioned remedy which I relearned from my father and I was very tempted to try again. This was to provide the sheep with troughs of treacle or crude molasses. Sheep love treacle and it is a very good source of energy, and father never had any more trouble with Toxaemia after he hit upon this idea. He did have to learn, however, to take the troughs away after the sheep had lambed, as lambs were forever getting stuck in the stuff, and tragically one year a lamb became so enmeshed in the sticky mess that it died, choked by treacle.

With good luck and especially good management, the flock and its keepers arrive at lambing time, whether it is in the depths of winter in a cosy shed, or on a hillside in April/May time, with the prospect of the generation of another years' lambs. This has to be the most satisfying time for anyone dealing with sheep.

Ewes that are lambed in shed, open yards or "in bye" fields (that is one close to the farm), are watched over very closely day and night. Those farmers with enough sheep to justify it, will have evolved a system for the maternity ward where each person will work an eight hour shift in 24 hours. This is necessary for two reasons; the obvious is that if a sheep is having difficulties in giving birth she may need assistance from the shepherd. If for whatever reason the shepherd or shepherdess (and I find in this context that women are better than men), cannot cope, they will at this point call in the veterinary surgeon. The other less obvious reason for close supervision at this time is the need to ensure that the mother has her own lambs! When two or more sheep lamb at the same time, the possible permutation of offspring are endless. Some ewes will happily give her lambs away to another who may want at least six offspring before she has even lambed! The answer is to ensure that when birth takes place, mother and child are placed in a small bonding pen to make sure they get to know each other, and that the lambs are sucking and getting the proper maternal attention. When the bonding process is complete, normally in no more than a day or two, the family can be allowed out, usually into a field with some shelter, and mother and children know each other in among hundreds without any possibility of a mistake. This recognition is done by a mixture of voice and smell, with the latter being the most important factor. Occasionally it is necessary to foster a lamb onto another mother, perhaps because her lamb has died and another ewe has triplets. This fostering process is accomplished by skinning the dead lamb, and putting its coat over the foster lamb. The ewe may take a day or two to be reconciled to her new baby, but it usually works in the end.

Many farmers in business in a smaller way have to cope with lambing by themselves, and an exhausting job it is. Most will work almost a 24 hour day, checking their mothers to be every few hours through the night, and cat napping in the farm kitchen or in a caravan or shed in the lambing field in between births. My father used to spend his nights going out to the sheep and in between times tying fishing flies at the kitchen table. If the weather was bad he would probably have a hypothermic lamb warming up in the oven of the range at the same time!

For the veterinary surgeon, lambing time also means a time of ever increasing activity as any difficulties that cannot be resolved by the shepherd and his helpers will these days find their way to the surgery in the back of a landrover or truck. It's not unusual at busy times to have a queue forming, and there is often the necessity of quickly sorting the emergency from the less urgent. This often requires diplomacy as the farmer often rightly sees his case as requiring the most immediate attention.

Many of the obstetrical difficulties can only be resolved by doing a caesarean operation on the ewe, and this is an operation that can become almost routine, especially in the surgery operating theatre. Most of these operations are performed with the sheep being given a local anaesthetic only, and it is not unusual for the ewe to be eating hay throughout the procedure.

Routine it may become, but there is little to compare with the sight of a mother with lambs after a successful operation, and the lambs nuzzling in to get their first important drink of colostrum. It even compensates for getting out of a warm bed on a cold winter night.

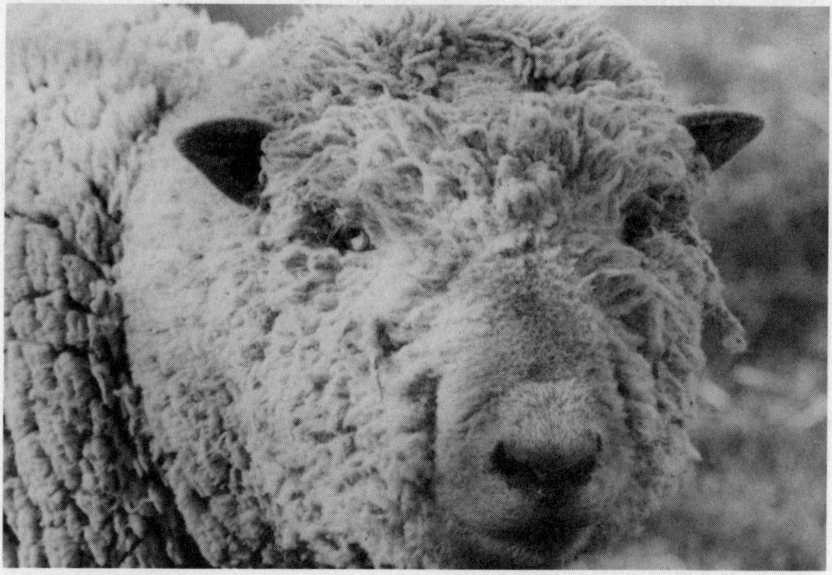

"Joly", the Southdown Ram — looking forward to seeing your ewes soon!

ONLY FOOLS AND HORSES

I suppose at the outset, I ought to apologise for the title of this chapter, but I've had a bad day so the title must stand! Besides, the reason for my bad temper was yet another example of how some people through their own thoughtlessness cause untold suffering to animals.

The case I had attended reminded me of so many others where much pain to horses and grief to the owners could so easily have been avoided by routine preventative measures. Take tetanus as an example. I still remember my first clinical case of tetanus in a horse. It was in a two year old part bred Arab filly, she was beautiful; and unvaccinated.

I was called to see her in the afternoon and found no external signs of injury, but she did have early signs of tetanus. She was frightened, stiff, trembling, running a temperature and beginning to dribble from the mouth. I gave her massive dosses of penicillin, intravenous antitetanus serum and a sedative. This constitutes the standard treatment for tetanus which has changed little over the years, but I came away from her with no sense other than one of acute foreboding for her welfare.

An early visit the next day confirmed all of my worst fears. She was dying with all the horrors of the disease. She was on her side but partially propped up against a bale of straw which was knocked away every time she had a convulsion. Unable to swallow due to the "lock jaw" she looked terrified, and I put her out of her misery as soon as I possibly could.

Her owners were very distressed, and quite unable to understand how she could have tetanus without any obvious external signs of injury. They had believed, like many others, that it was all right to leave tetanus vaccination injections until the animal has an injury. Or it may have been the syndrome of "it can't happen to us" working again. It only takes a scratch, perhaps a thorn penetrating somewhere, or a cut in the gum for the tetanus bacillus to enter the tissues and the poison spread through the body. The tetanus germs are all around, in the soil, and are particularly prevalent where horses are grazing. Horses and ponies apparently pass thousands of these bacteria in their dung every day. It makes no sense not to protect the animal as even today, with all the modern treatments and drugs that are available, still only one case in ten will survive clinical symptoms - if you are lucky.

There are many other equine disorders which can be just as easily prevented as tetanus. That other common condition, colic, which most of the horse and pony owning public dreads above any others, can be prevented, usually by the most simple precautions. Colic is a symptom, not a disease entity in itself, and means that the animal is suffering abdominal pain. Many colics are the result of constipation, dental disorders or internal parasites. During winter months, colic due to constipation is a great nuisance, mostly as the result of the animal gorging on its straw bedding, or by simple fault in its feeding. Constipation can be easily prevented by putting the horse on a bed of wood shavings, peat moss or even shredded paper. However, if the owner wants to continue bedding on straw and if the animal is on a farm where there is a super abundance of the material, who can blame them - the remedy is straightforward enough. All that needs to be done is to put a scoop of unfashionable bran or mollassed chaff in the feed daily, or better still feed a good bran mash two to three times a week.

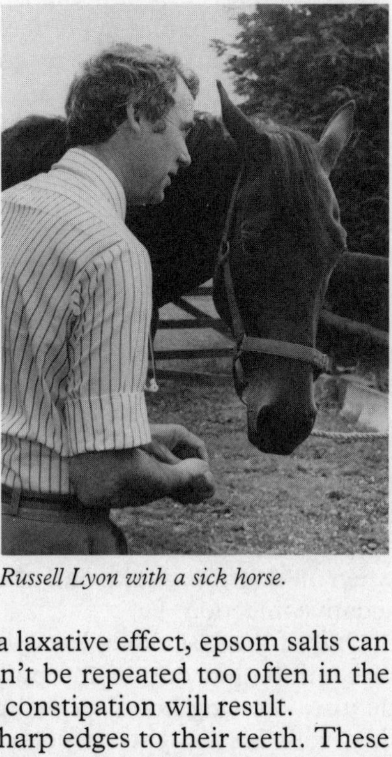

Anna Oakford

Russell Lyon with a sick horse.

Too many people nowadays don't seem to know how to make a proper bran mash. Giving a recipe will make me sound a bit like Delia Smith but no matter for that.

Depending on the size of the animal, put two to four pounds of bran in a bucket with one to two tablespoons of ordinary salt. Add enough boiling water to damp the whole and stir well. Cover it and allow to steam for about fifteen minutes and it should then be cool enough for the horse to eat. For extra laxative effect, epsom salts can be substituted for salt, but it shouldn't be repeated too often in the week as the rather opposite effect to constipation will result.

Most horses and ponies develop sharp edges to their teeth. These sharp points are usually found on the outer edge of the top molars and the inner edge of the bottom teeth. These can be fairly easily detected by the vet or an experienced horse person. An inexperienced groom putting their fingers in a horse's mouth to check the molars in quite liable to get their fingers badly bitten! However, if a horse or pony is dropping food from its mouth while eating, then it's a fairly safe bet that something is hurting in its mouth, and it's usually the teeth.

The point of all this activity in the mouth and the prevention of colic is that if a horse can't chew properly because of soreness, then it is liable to bolt its food which can lead to digestive disorders which in turn lead to colic. I tend to tell clients that most of their animals will need their teeth checking once or twice a year. If they are found to be in need of attention then the sharp bits are rasped or filed down by an instrument particularly made for the job. Most vets have evolved their own way of doing this. If the patient is fairly quiet, I find all that is required by way of restraining the horse is for the handler to hold the animal's tongue out of the side of its mouth. This then allows me to file down the teeth on the opposite side without the tongue getting in the way.

Occasionally a mouth gag is required as well to keep the mouth open, as some (ponies in particular) are very adept at biting the tooth instrument and stopping any further progress! Animals that resent the procedure, and there are quite a few that do, may require twitching. Often to a lay person this seems a barbarous thing to do to any animal, and I must admit I used to agree. Twitching involves putting a piece of cord on the end of the horse's nose, then twisting it tight with a piece of wood to which the cord is attached. Doing this, nine times out of ten, stops any misbehaviour and the job can be done. I used to believe that it worked by giving the horse an alternative pain to think about, but I couldn't quite reconcile that opinion with the average horse's demeanour when the twitch is applied. They tend to behave almost as if in a trance.

Recent scientific work has shown that the end of the nose is an acupuncture point. Stimulation of that point causes the release of endorphines (which are natural pain killers produced by the body) into the system, and goes a long way to explaining why a correctly applied twitch causes the effect it does. Of course there are times when it doesn't work, and then I resort to giving the animal a sedative injection.

One of the last times I was in the dentist's chair, I found to my discomfort that one of my molars required filing down a bit. My dentist, knowing how I rasped down ponies teeth, as I have had to deal with his daughter's ponies, threatened to treat me in a like manner! I think he meant pulling my tongue out to the side as I couldn't see a twitch in his dental armoury (although I often think the suction apparatus is an adequate substitute), but he had me worried for a moment.

Not so very long ago I had a one ton shire stallion as a patient, in the prime of its life, killed by a worm less than half an inch long in its adult form. How can this happen? The animals on that farm had all been dewormed regularly but unfortunately not regularly enough, and red worm larvae had migrated through the animal's body and penetrated the blood vessels that supply the bowel. This caused an aneurysm, or blockage in the blood supply, which resulted in a spasm in the bowel and then colic. When an animal has a pain in its belly its first instinct is to lie down and then roll, and this is just what the stallion did. Almost immediately, the gut became twisted from the rolling - and the colic became a killer colic. When this happens and the diagnosis is made quickly, there is a chance for the horse if it can be operated on without undue delay. We in East Anglia are so fortunate to be living near that centre of excellence for horses - Newmarket. Help from colleagues with equine hospital facilities is just a phone call away day or night. It is then just a matter of transporting the patient there, sometimes not that easy, and leaving it in the experts' capable hands. However, even in the best of circumstances there is still only a success rate of about fifty percent, if you are one of the lucky ones, and I'm sad to say this particular stallion didn't make it. Another consideration for the owner is the cost of abdominal surgery which can be easily over two thousand pounds whether the animal lives or dies. And all this can often be avoided by deworming regularly every four to six weeks for the cost of a few pounds only.

Most horse disorders like the ones just mentioned are the result of domestication. Laminitis is a prime example of this. This is a condition which affects the lamina of the feet. The lamina is the spongy part of the foot between the pedal bone and the hard outer wall of the foot. Affected animals are often in acute pain which in some cases can be very difficult to control. Typically the horse or pony will stand in a rocking horse type position, trying to take as much pressure as possible off the front feet which are usually affected most severely. If the animal moves at all, it is very haltingly and then it tends to shuffle around like an old man wearing ill fitting slippers. I sometimes describe the pain that I think the animal may be suffering from as equivalent to that which we feel when we hit ourselves on the nail with a hammer. Bleeding occurs under the nail and it can be excruciatingly painful. How much worse must it be for the horse having to stand on feet when they are hurting to that degree. Laminitis is mostly the result of bad management by the owner and is commonly seen in over-weight ponies that have been allowed to stuff themselves on grass. This usually happens in the spring when the grass is very rich and at its most lush. It also tends to coincide with the end of the school holiday. If a pony is exercised regularly, then a reasonable diet is required to give it the energy to keep it going. If, however, it is allowed to eat the same when school has started and it's not getting the same amount of work, then it will get too fat and laminitis will result. Although the disease can be caused by other things such as womb infections after foaling, by far the likeliest reason is over feeding, which just a little foresight and common sense can overcome. Not that the average owner is totally to blame; there is still an insistence by many show judges for horses to be shown too fat. If they are not in "show condition" (which is too fat), then they have no chance of rosettes let alone winning. The outcome of the illness in some severe cases can be fatal. Damage to the lamina, if profound, can result in the pedal bone (which is the bone within the hoof), coming through the sole of the foot. Even today this can mean the animal having to be destroyed to stop it suffering uncontrollable pain.

Recent research into the subject has changed quite markedly the way vets now treat laminitis. It was thought that standing a patient with sore feet in cold running water did much to alleviate the pain. This is now known to be quite the wrong thing to do. The patient has a much better chance of pain relief, despite the feet being warm to touch, if the feet are immersed in warm water.

The cold water treatment is now as out of date as bleeding the patient. Bleeding a horse which had laminitis used to be common practice. It was done by using a fleam or bleeding knife which was tapped into the animals jugular vein, and two or three pints of blood would be removed. It was thought that as this would reduce the patients blood pressure albeit for a transitory period, some pain relief would be obtained. Now drugs are used to improve the blood's circulation within the foot and this has proved to be a great benefit to the patients.

Asthma is an increasingly common disorder in people, as I know to my cost within my own family. What is not generally realised is that horses can get asthma too, but it is given a much grander name; Chronic Obstructive Pulmonary Disease or C.O.P.D. for short. This disease in horse is, like that in people, increasingly seen. I cannot help feeling that this increased incidence can not be only due to improved diagnosis, but may also have something to do with the increasing level of pollution in the atmosphere.

What is certain is that the disease has been documented in equines for many centuries and was called Broken Wind or Heaves. These descriptions speak for themselves. The animal, often over a period of months, gradually and slowly loses lung function. This is accompanied by an increased respiratory rate and persistent dry cough. It can also, in another form, have a sudden onset, where the animal can become very distressed over short periods of time, and in some cases die. Most of the time horses and ponies with C.O.P.D. are allergic to stable dust and the component of this that causes most of the trouble is the fungal spores which are found even in the best hay. Mild cases can be easily and quickly cured. They are just turned out in the fresh air, and care must be taken not to feed them dry hay. If it's winter time and they are not a tough breed used to the outdoor life, they have to be provided with a water proof coat called a New Zealand Rug and a field shelter. If it's summer, then some shade from the sun will do. If hay has to be fed, it must be soaked before feeding. A thirty minute immersion of the hay net in a tub of water is all that is required to denature the fungal spores and render them innocuous. A good hay equivalent is now available commercially in sealed bags, it comes under a variety of brand names including "Horsehage". It looks and smells like silage that cows get to eat, and it is just wilted grass of a good type, packed into a polythene hag. Horses love it, and can easily eat their daily ration in a very short space of time. This is a bit of a drawback if the animal is stabled as it then gets easily bored having nothing else to do! By contrast, a hay net can take some time to munch through. If it is not practical to keep the affected animals outdoors all the time, then the stable must be thoroughly cleansed down to get rid of all dust particles and cobwebs. This is usually managed with a pressure water hose or an industrial vacuum cleaner. When this is done then the ventilation has got to be looked at in the stable, as far too many have inadequate airflows through them. The traditional half door left open is not good enough.

If the stable box is in line with others, sharing a common air space, then like measures have to be taken in them as well. Now that the cause of C.O.P.D. has become more understood, so more new drugs have become available to treat the illness.

Clenbuterol is a drug used in human medicine and works very well in horses, as does the inhalant drug cromoglycate, first used to treat asthma in people. A horse can be induced to inhale a medicine quite easily. A bag not unlike the old fashioned nose feed bag is placed over the animal's muzzle and made to fit tightly to the animals facial contours. The drug is then introduced into the bag by means of a hand or foot pump, and this makes it impossible for the patient to do anything other than breathe in the medication. Most of the horses do, with remarkably good grace considering that it must be a pretty frightening experience, at least for the first few times. An inhalation two to three times a week is usually enough to keep the condition at bay.

I hope it will be apparent from the foregoing, that many horse ailments are the result of man's interference and ignorance of what enables a horse to enjoy a healthy lifestyle. Prevention, as has been said many times, is better than cure. In many cases the prevention that is required is a little thought and knowledge, but if it does occasionally mean spending a bit of money, that will still be cheaper than attempting a cure once the animal is ill.

Talking of money leads me on to a seemingly unrelated subject of insurance.. More and more of the horse and pet owning public are aware of the benefits of insurance to pay for the vet bills or if the worst comes to the worse, a new horse. Insurance today is not cheap, and I know that many people don't insure because of the cost. However, there is one type of insurance that every one should have if they have animals, and that is third party cover. It is extremely foolish not have this basic protection.

It's all too easy, even with the best of fences for horses and dogs as well to get out and stray onto the road with disastrous consequences both for animals and people. The sight of a dead horse on the road as a result of it straying into the path of car in the pitch dark is not pleasant. If there are human casualties it is even worse. If it's your animal that's involved, and you are at fault, then you could be liable to considerable damages claims.

On the positive side, many people have third party cover without being aware of the fact as it is often included in a good house insurance policy. If it is not, then such cover can be arranged for very little cost.

A client recently was faced with the nightmare of her horse causing a serious accident. She thought she was not insured and was faced with a bill for many thousands of pounds. You can imagine her relief to discover that her house insurance policy covered that type of accident. It didn't pay for a new horse, but it helped to assuage the loss more than a little.

I have written at some length about the foolishness of some owners but I am at the same time very aware that animals can make fools of us all, not least the veterinary surgeon. I have only to remind myself of a recent case where, with great regret I pronounced that the patient, a Percheron stallion of some antiquity, would be extremely unlikely to rise again. He had an operation to remove a cancerous testicle which was a success, but when he was given the antidote to the anaesthetic he was quite unable to get to his feet.

A colleague went on my behalf a few hours later and gave him another stimulant drug normally only given to small animals. Samson then leapt to his feet and now, a few months on, positively gleams with health and may yet sire another foal this season!

THE OFFICIAL VETERINARY SURGEON

Most veterinary surgeons in private practice are called on from time to time to act in some official capacity in one way or another. For example, many vets in agricultural or mixed practice are part time veterinary officers for the Ministry of Agriculture, Fisheries and Food. As such the private vet has had a large responsibility for the control and eradication of many notifiable diseases. Diseases such as Tuberculous, Brucellosis and Anthrax are the subject of legislation. This means that if a farmer or stockperson suspects the presence of these diseases (or others on the list of notifiable diseases), then they must by law inform the police or the local divisional veterinary officer of their suspicions. Failure to do this can result in prosecution.

In most cases, full time officers from the Ministry will take charge of the operation to control and eradicate the outbreak of disease. There have been many occasions in the past, however, when due to lack of personnel, private vets have to be used to augment the full time officers. The last time this happened to any extent was during the Foot and Mouth outbreak in the late 1960's, when many vets were drafted to help control the disease. Apart from this "fire brigade role" at a time of crisis, much of the day to day responsibility for the control of long standing, endemic, notifiable diseases like Tuberculous or Brucellosis, devolves to the local vet.

Every month most mixed practices are sent lists of farms where the animals have to be tested on a yearly to two yearly basis for those two infections. Tuberculous used to be a terrible scourge of animals and man in this country. The most likely cause of TB in people used to be by infection directly from the cattle, or indirectly by drinking infected milk. Now, with the disease under control (apart from some farms in the south west) and with the pasteurisation of milk, this risk to man has all but disappeared. Nowadays, if a cow is found to have tuberculosis, it is much more likely that the herdsman has infected the cow rather than the other way!

Routine testing of cattle has brought about this change of affairs over the last half century. All cattle are subjected to an intra dermal test. The skin of the neck is clipped in two places, above and below each other, and the thickness of the skin is measured with callipers. A very small amount (0.1ml) of killed avaian tuberculin and killed bovine tuberculin is injected into the skin at the prepared sites. The tuberculin has to be killed otherwise it would infect the animal. The cattle are re-examined three days later when the skin thickness is measured again. If the skin reaction on the bovine site is greater than the avian site then the beast may well have tuberculosis and have to be slaughtered. The farmer is compensated for any that have to be killed for this reason, and then much work has to be done by the Ministry vets to try and trace the source of the outbreak.

It is by these means that TB has been virtually eradicated, except for a few isolated pockets in the country where the cattle seem to become re-infected by the badger population. It is still proving to be quite a headache to control the disease in badgers, and attempts to limit the spread of infection by killing badgers in known infected badger sets, seem to have gone disastrously wrong in some cases. There are hopes, however, that it may be possible to vaccinate the badger against the disease. An oral vaccine put into bait which the animal will eat, may be the best way forward.

Brucellosis is another notifiable disease which has been largely wiped out over the last twenty years. The disease causes abortion in cattle and undulant fever in man. It is a bacterial infection which is particularly nasty in people, as it causes a high temperature, and a malaise that can go on for months, and quite a few of my colleagues have suffered from its effects over the years. Indeed, a partner from my practice had to take premature retirement due to this illness.

The test of the disease in cattle is very straight-forward and only involves taking a blood sample which is then submitted to the Central Laboratory in Weybridge. The results, if positive, will mean the infected animal having to be culled from the herd, again with compensation.

These two diseases are only an example of the many other infectious diseases which we have to deal with as official vets. There are some like Foot and Mouth disease, Swine Fever and Rabies which are not present in the UK at the moment. But this doesn't mean they won't be back, and we as a profession must keep up our guard at all times against any possibility of fresh outbreaks.

The chance of Rabies arriving again in this country and becoming endemic in the wildlife fills me with horror. A walk or a picnic in the countryside would never by the same again if all the time we had to be on our guard against rabid animals. Contrary to what most people think, a fox for example, infected with Rabies would be unlikely to rush out from the undergrowth, foaming at the mouth. It is much more likely to have the dumb form of the disease, where it loses all fear of people, and could easily be fondled by a child. That is why I feel we must keep up our quarantine restrictions on dogs, cats, small animals like guinea pigs and rats, as well as primates, despite pressure from

Common Market countries, among others, to lower our frontiers.

All animals entering quarantine premises for the mandatory six months, have to be vaccinated against rabies, and are inspected by an official veterinary surgeon every day (apart from Sundays and Bank Holidays) for any signs of the infection. If an animal dies while still in quarantine its brain has to be examined for any evidence of the virus which causes the disease. There is a good vaccination against Rabies, but once clinical symptoms appear there is no cure for the sufferer, whether animal or man, and they die in a horrible way.

There are many other duties and diseases which the local veterinary inspector has to be involved with, about which the public is largely unaware. Vets have to be involved with meat inspection, to ensure that the meat reaching the table is fit to eat.

Animals being exported to any part of the world have to be certified as healthy and fit to travel. All livestock markets have to be under veterinary supervision to make sure that any animal entering the market is fit to be there, fit to travel and demonstrates no clinical signs of any notifiable disease. To enable private vets to carry out all these duties, we have to be licensed by the Ministry of Agriculture and have a warrant card to produce when necessary. This allows us to enter premises and take such samples as are thought to be required for the purpose of examining and treating suspect animals. More strangely, we are given the authority to dig up (notwithstanding the Animal Health Act of 1984 which prohibits this), any carcass or part of carcass which is thought expedient to determine the cause of death.

Other "official" occasions for the local vet include attendance, usually in a honorary capacity, at the local agricultural show. This is, unless the vet has particular expertise with other animals, to help either with judging horse classes or dogs and cats, or to measure the height of the ponies for the different classes. This last procedure is usually farcical as an animal has to be fairly relaxed and unworried to get fair indication of its height! This is something that is well nigh impossible to achieve if the measuring pad on the showground is in view of any other livestock.

As a young vet I approached these local shows with some misgivings, not to say trepidation, believing in all the horror stories of the pitfalls that await the inexperienced. My senior partner helped to calm my fears and to put me right in many ways, but the vet who helped me most in this respect lived and worked in the neighbouring town.

He was one of the finest clinicians and veterinary surgeons of the old school that I had the privilege of knowing, and he died only a few years ago. He was not a man to suffer fools gladly, but he often went out of his way to explain and help the genuine owner or colleague who sought his assistance and advice. Nor was he over ready to send in a bill, which endeared him to many more people!

There is a wealth of stories and legends told about him, probably mostly apocryphal, but some must be true, and I can vouch for the following.

Many years ago, the most popular entertainment at agricultural shows, apart from the displays of livestock and the beer tent, was the trotting races. These races were usually held after the grand parade of prize winners, from the middle of the afternoon until the show closed. This activity has largely been superseded by show jumping, which I think is a much inferior spectator sport.

The organising committee of the show would hire a promoter who would turn up on the appointed afternoon with the necessary horses, jockeys and all the other required accoutrements, and races would be run. It was always a splendid spectacle with much noise and colour, dust and mud flying everywhere, depending on the whim of the weather. It always evoked memories of "Ben Hur" or the "Calgary Stampede" on impressionable spectators like myself!

I do suspect the main reason for the popularity of the event was the opportunity it afforded the members of the public to bet on the outcome of each race. Why this should be the case I have never quite been able to fathom, as I always understood that the bookmakers were hand in glove with the promoter. There was very little profit to be had, except for those "in the know".

Joe Brown (not his real name but it will suffice) had for many years been the honourary veterinary surgeon to the show. All this meant was that he would be present all day and attend to animals that required attention, and if he was lucky he would get a free lunch and a drink for his trouble.

One particular show afternoon, after the first race, one of the horses sustained a cut on its leg, and a request was made for veterinary assistance. Joe was called and examined the animal to find that it required a few stitches in the wound. This was duly done and the grateful promoter asked Joe how much he owed him.

"Oh no," came the reply, "I am proud to be the honorary veterinary surgeon to the show, and as such I am only too pleased and happy to do this job free of charge, however," he continued, sotto voice, "if you would like to give your opinion as to who might win the next race?" He left the aside in the air, and was duly and discreetly rewarded with a name.

That race was soon over and after Joe had collected his winnings from the bookmaker, he had a further thought that perhaps he ought to administer an anti-tetanus injection to the injured horse. He checked the animal again, and after giving the injection was again asked by a very pleased and gratified promoter as to his fee for services rendered. The reply was the same as the previous time.

"I wouldn't hear of charging you for this as you know I am honorary veterinary surgeon to the show, and I am only too pleased to do this for your horse." He let the aside go by this time, but received the owner's tip again. The afternoon proceeded in a like manner to everyone's satisfaction, and further frequent visits were made to make sure that the patient was well. Such going's on wouldn't happen nowadays, but it all happened a long time ago, and no one thought it strange or wrong at the time.

Vets have to be in attendance at all horse race meetings and also at greyhound racing tracks, where these are under the control of the National Greyhound Racing Association. As official vet at a racing track, one's behaviour has to above suspicion and reproach. As a matter of course, all staff are disallowed to bet on the outcome of any race, in case they may be tempted to take some action that may alter the outcome of race.

Until fairly recently my practice attended at a local greyhound track on a regular basis, and our duties as vets started at about 6.30 in the evening. This involved checking in all dogs that were due to run during the evening.

There were usually about sixty runners all together, and they all had to be examined to make sure they were not lame, and were in a fit state to run. This had to be done between 6.30pm and 7.15pm as the first race started at 7.30pm. As well as the veterinary inspection, the dogs had to be weighed and positively identified before they were locked into individual kennels until it was their turn.

The reason for all this checking was and is to try and ensure that all races were fair and above board, with no dogs subjected to any activity which would enhance or detract from this performance. Or in other words to prevent "nobbling".

Over the years the general public's perception of greyhound racing is that much of it is blemished by owners or trainers, or some other outsiders with betting interests doping the dogs to alter their racing performance. While this is by no means as common as many think, tampering still goes on.

A common method of doing this is to reduce the dog's performance by some means over a few races, and then when the chosen race comes along the dog is allowed to run to its true potential. This can be done quite easily, without using drugs, by altering some part of its training or feeding schedule. The racing odds on a dog having had a few poor performances are good, therefore when it unexpectedly wins, a lot of money can be made from the "bookie".

Naturally when a dog unexpectedly runs well or poorly, questions are asked and very often samples are taken for drug testing. Anyone found guilty of a misdemeanour in this way will be banned from the track, and trainers banned from training by the National Greyhound Racing Association.

I must emphasise again, in case I give a thoroughly wrong impression, that the majority of owners and trainers are very honest and would not be involved in any illegal schemes, particularly where it may harm their charges.

However, despite the risks to man and dogs "nobbling" still goes on occasionally, particularly on unlicensed (flapping) tracks. The last method of stopping, that is to say slowing a dog, that I encountered while I was still officiating, was to spray a flea spray aerosol through the mesh grill of the animal's kennel after it had been inspected. In the narrow confines of the kennel this adversely affects the atmosphere and the dog's performance is slightly impaired. This method is virtually impossible to prove unless you catch someone in the act, as most greyhounds have to be treated regularly for fleas anyway. Eternal vigilance is the only way to try and combat the cheat, but every now and again the unexpected can happen - and one night it did.

It was a big race night, there was a large crowd, the stadium was buzzing with a barely suppressed excitement and activity which increased to a fever pitch as it got nearer to the main event of the evening; the area final. There was a lot of money at stake, both in prizes and with the bookmakers.

After each race is run the security steward has to walk around the perimeter of the track to make sure that all is well and safe before the next race. He particularly makes sure that the perimeter fence is secure, in this case a corrugated iron fence. His final task before the next race is to replace the mechanical hare (known in all greyhound circles as the "bunny"), on the running rail and to get it into position ready for the off.

The dogs were paraded in front of the grandstand as usual and then loaded into the starting traps. The starter checked to see that all was well and set the hare off on the rail. When it passed the traps the dogs were released, the crowd roared and the race was on. The runners had to go twice around the track but halfway round the second circuit the race came to a shuddering and confused halt as the "bunny" fell off its rail!

The story of the technical problem was explained a little later. Apparently the wrong dog had been winning the race, from a betting syndicate's point of view, and a signal had gone out from somewhere in the grandstand to an accomplice, who was hiding behind the corrugated fence for just such an emergency. At the agreed signal he thrust a stick through a convenient hole and knocked the hare off the rail as it passed.

The race had to be declared null and void, to be run again at some other time and all bets had to be returned. The guilty parties were suspected but never found, and forever after that night is remembered as the night the hare was nobbled and not a dog!

For a private veterinary surgeon being an "official" vet is often thought to be the dull, less interesting side of practice, but in my experience, it has its moments as well!

MUTILATIONS OR THE THINGS WE DO TO ANIMALS

From the time that stone age man changed from being a hunter of animals to herding them instead, he tried to make them more amenable to domestication. Those nomadic herders must have realised very early on that a castrated animal is much easier to domesticate than an entire one. How right they were! However, in these more enlightened times,in this country at least, castration is realised to be a mutilation and should be avoided wherever possible in farm animals.

Although it's impossible to say, it is quite likely that horses were the first large animals to be tamed and castrated by man. This would depend to some extent on what they were being used for: to be kept for meat and transport, a quiet sensible beast is a necessity, but for war, stallions were regarded as highly desirable for the cavalry soldier. The Romans in particular knew the advantages to be had by riding a furious fighting stallion. They developed many fierce pieces of restraining equipment to control them, to the rider's advantage and the enemies' disadvantage. The Islamic culture actually banned the castration of horses on religious grounds.

The method of castrating equines has changed very little in essential details over the centuries. A study of Roman and Arabic texts proves this very readily. Basically, the animal has to be restrained in such a way to enable the operator to make two incisions into the scrotum and remove both testicles. A method of staunching the bleeding had to be used, and much skill would be required by the operator to avoid injury to himself, and serious consequences to the patient.

When I first became a veterinary surgeon, the method used by the practice that I joined was very old fashioned, but safe and effective. The animal was twitched to restrain it (as previously described in an earlier chapter), and given a sedative injection into the jugular vein. This usually worked quite quickly and then allowed the vet to inject local anaesthetic into the animal's scrotum. Then came the dangerous bit! The operation was carried out with the horse standing and the vet crouched to one side, and halfway under the patient's belly to carry out the necessary incisions. You can well imagine the difficult and dangerous position this was for the vet, despite the horse being sedated, and the relevant area hopefully impervious to pain.

To stop any bleeding, clams were used. These are two pieces of wood about six inches long and about the thickness of a middle fingers, held together at one end by boiled string. The inner surface had a caustic ointment on it, known as a red blister. After the cuts were made, the clams were then placed on either side of the exposed blood vessels, and the ends not held by string were shut together by a small leather collar. The horse was then left like this for twenty four hours with the testicles hanging free under its belly, exposed to the elements. When the animal was revisited the next day, the now dried out testicles were removed without any risk of bleeding. It was a highly successful procedure, which has, with some additional refinements like sedative and local anaesthetic, been in use for many centuries. Both Roman and Arab horsemen used clams to stop bleeding, the only apparent difference was that they had to tie their patients up and cast them on the ground in order to operate.

Horses and ponies are still castrated with them standing, by vets who have almost universally abandoned clams and instead use an emasculator. This is an instrument which after the incisions are made, removes the testicles with a crushing action on the blood vessels, which stops heavy bleeding. Otherwise the operation is the same as previously described or clams.

However, in common with many other veterinary surgeons, I prefer to give my patients a general anaesthetic which renders them unconscious, and leaves them lying on the ground for the operation. As you will easily imagine, this enables the site for surgery to be cleaned properly and the operation to be carried out unhurriedly, with far less risk to the animal and vet. The blood vessels are ligated with absorbable material, like cat gut, and the area dusted with a wound dressing and fly repellent powder before the horse gets to its feet.

The anaesthetic I employ for the operation was originally developed for use in dart guns for immobilising wild animals like elephants. It's highly dangerous stuff to the human operator, but not to the animal. Very great care must be taken when handling the material not to spill any on human skin, and the vet must avoid accidental injection at all costs.

Veterinary surgeons have died after accidents with this drug. For this very reason I take a veterinary nurse with me, and she has the antidote to the drug ready in case of an accident! All of my nurses are trained in how to administer the antidote, but given all possible administration sites on the human body, not one of them will tell me their chosen place should such an opportunity arise!

The advantage of using this potentially dangerous drug is that it is very safe in horses, and they will not come round from the anaesthetic until they are given the antidote. This given into the vein, will have them on their feet and eating within two or three minutes. Nevertheless, it's always a relief when the patient is awake and on his feet, the operation complete and everybody well.

On one occasion when a pony came round, it blundered into Janet my nurse, and sent her flying. I helped her to her feet fearing the worst, as she had gone a very nasty grey colour.

Equilibrium was restored however, when we discovered that she had been deposited into a dung heap, bottom first! Much of the smelly wet compost was stuck to her rear end and I had to insist on the car windows being wide open all the way back to the surgery, and she had to sit on newspaper. It quite made up for all the threats of where she might inject any antidote into me!

As I have said, my patients are asleep and lying on the ground while I operate on them, and it is often difficult to find a suitable, clean, soft piece of earth on which to drop the horse. On one occasion I met a client at a location of his choice. It was in a lane where he said there was a good site for the procedure. As I followed the path, I soon found where he meant, it was at the local golf course. The ground beside the third tee was perfect and the fairway was deserted. The operation went like clockwork, with no hitches and fortunately no spectators. I did heave a large sigh of relief when it was all over, but on reflection I had to admit that it was the first, and I hope the last time, that I had taken two off on that particular par three hole!

Castrating cattle and sheep is a much easier procedure for all concerned. Up to seven days old a tight rubber ring can be placed around the neck of the scrotum. It causes the whole scrotal sack to slough off after a few days, and does a very effective job. Farmers and stockmen like this method as it is very simple, there is no blood, and very little risk to the patient. After more than seven days from birth, this procedure is not allowed as it is considered, quite rightly, too painful to be allowed on welfare grounds. Up to the age of two months, a farmer or shepherd is allowed to castrate a beast or lamb without anaesthetic, as it is recognised that giving a local anaesthetic can often be as painful as the operation itself. After two months of age, only a vet is allowed to carry out the procedure, and then only after giving an anaesthetic.

The basic method is the same as for horses, but haemostasis is not required to the same extent. After the cuts are made, if the testis and the blood vessels are extracted carefully and fully, then little bleeding occurs and no ligatures are required.

If it is summer time and there are flies about, with all the risk of maggot strike, then many people prefer to have their stock castrated with a burdizzo. This is an instrument invented by an Italian, which castrates the animal by crushing the spermatic cord and blood vessels. Deprived in this way of a blood supply, the testicles wither away in a few weeks. The burdizzo was invented for use in the tropics, but it has been of much use in this country as well. I personally don't like using it as I think they cause more post operative pain than the simple surgical operation.

It used to be a common practice among farmers in Scotland to castrate ram lambs with their teeth! My father used this technique every year, and what's more it was a method that made some sense. The lambs were held in such a way that they couldn't struggle, with their backsides on the top rail of the sheep pen, belly turned towards the operator. The "surgeon" would make the necessary cuts with a sharp knife and then extract the testicles with his teeth. It was done in this way as invariably the shepherd's mouth was cleaner than his hands, and therefore reduced the risk of infection to the sheep by a considerable amount.

I had a gym teacher who always pestered me to bring him the testicles when the lambs were being "cut". I had to take a bag of the offending bits to school for his delectation. He liked them fried! He was a great bully of a man, and my secret revenge was never to tell him how the job was done!

Dad carried on this way with the lambs for many years, and only stopped when he had to have dentures. He just couldn't do the job without his own teeth.

We, and the animals under our care are fortunate that the practice of castrating meat animals is slowly dying out. Pigs are hardly ever castrated now, as with improved husbandry the pigs are ready for market before the meat becomes tainted by the smell of male hormone. This is also the case with beef cattle. I am pleasantly relieve by this, as I tend to have a belief in reincarnation which was disturbed by the thought that if there was any justice in this world, after all the pigs I had "cut" my fate would be to be reborn as a hog pig that had to be castrated!

Dogs and cats have long been required to have a general anaesthetic before they are allowed to be neutered, but it wasn't always the case. As a young lad I witnessed, on a fairly remote hill farm, a cat castration without any anaesthetic at all. The victim was stuffed head first into a Wellington boot. The scrotum was then snipped and the testicles extracted, to the accompanying screeches of the unfortunate animal. When he was released from the boot, he shot off at great speed up the hill, and I doubt if he ventured down again for some time. How glad I am that we are now finished with such barbarities.

Tail docking is a mutilation for which there can be little justification, except on health grounds. Up until the late 1940's horses, and in particular heavy working horses, had their tails docked because it was a fashionable thing to do. No consideration was given to the horse that it just might have a need of a tail to keep the flies away, and for protection of a very sensitive area.

The operation was carried out by a veterinary surgeon who had to be very skilled and quick on his feet as no anaesthetics were used. The "real" experts reckoned to do the job with a single flash of the scalpel, having first located the appropriate gap in the tail vertebrae. Those not so skilled would use a docking knife, which looks like a portable guillotine, to chop the tail off.

Bleeding was stopped by using either a pine tar compound or cautery, or even by using what was left of the tail hairs to weave a matrix of material over the stump. This last method helped to clot the blood more readily.

I am told that most vets were highly relieved when legislation brought about the end of this abhorrent business, and I often feel that it was a great pity that the legislators didn't outlaw docking of puppy tails at the same time. This procedure has only now been stopped since the beginning of July 1993 when it became illegal for any lay person to cut off puppy dogs tails. The Royal College of Veterinary Surgeons has stated that the docking of dogs' tails by a vet, other than for therapeutic reasons, will now be grounds for that vet to be struck off as one of their members, thus disbarring the vet from practising as a veterinary surgeon. This will be done on the grounds of disgraceful and unprofessional conduct. Most vets have heaved a collective sigh of relief, as it was one of the most unpleasant jobs we had to do.

I made a habit for some years that when I docked tails I had the owner present to hold the little creature, and observe just what they were putting it through. When the scissors started cutting and the blood was running, it was not uncommon that only the first one or two was done. The owner, if not a regular breeder and hardened to it, would stop the proceedings and leave the rest as nature intended.

Docking had been allowed to continue for so many years after being stopped in horses, as there was and still is a very strong lobby in favour of the practice. This lobby was supported by many in the Kennel Club and by some veterinary surgeons. It has been argued that game dogs will be very liable to get their tails lacerated when running into rough scrub and woodland in the pursuit of game. I can't go along with this myself as it doesn't seem to affect foxes or hounds, and I can't remember having a retriever, which is an undocked breed, damaging its tail in this way.

Every dog needs a tail for balance and to express itself, and I do hope that given time even the most die-hard in the dog world will come to recognise that the bad practice which they have supported, over too many years, was only dictated by fashion and that all dogs look much better with their tails left on.

Many intensive pig units have to dock piglets tails to reduce the risk of tail biting in later life. This vice is a result of stressful living conditions, and it would be better all round to try and alleviate the causes of the vice, such as overcrowding rather than resorting to the simple expedient of chopping a tail off.

The docking of any pig over seven days old is prohibited except when performed by a vet, and then only for health reasons. The one group of animals in which it is necessary to dock tails is sheep. It is easy to justify this operation in lambs for therapeutic reasons as undocked lambs are far more likely to be struck by blowflies and have maggots in their flesh. The tails are usually removed at the time of castration either by rubber ring or knife. Care must be taken not to cut the tail too short as it must be allowed to cover the sensitive area of the back passage and the vulval region in females. It is a welfare offence to cut the tail too short.

At the time when horse docking was banned, ear cropping in dogs was also banned. This is a practice which is still carried out in the United States and parts of Europe. What happens is that under a general anaesthetic the dogs ears are trimmed and in some cases shortened in order that the ears permanently stand up, giving the animal a permanently alert expression. It is mostly done to Great Dane, Boxers and Dobermans and it is still not uncommon to get requests for the operation to be performed on puppies from these breeds.

Some years ago a client was very persistent in his wish to have his new puppy attended to in this way. He was refused by every vet he approached in this country, so he sent the pup at the age of only eight weeks to Holland, where the operation was performed quite legally. The little creature was then brought back into this country where it had to undergo the normal period of quarantine for six months. This meant isolation for the animal at a most critical time of its young life. However, as the ears needed daily dressing (they had become infected) he received lots of attention and soon became a firm favourite with the kennel staff.

All attempts to turn him into a guard dog when he came out of quarantine came to nothing, as by that time having had so much attention, he thought every human was his friend! The expense involved in the exercise must have been considerable, and it was all for appearances sake and without a thought for the dog's well being.

One type of mutilation that I trust will never be banned, is dehorning. Failure to do this can result in cattle severely damaging each other by fighting and bullying. Quite recently a client of mine had a lovely Arab mare killed by a bull's horn in the ribs. It was a breakdown in management but it couldn't have happened had the bull already been dehorned. It's also a lot safer for the stockmen if they are looking after hornless animals.

It is common practice to remove the horn buds from goats and calves while they are still young. It is far less stressful to the animal to disbud at an early age as inevitably when older it is a bigger operation with a lot more difficulties involved in restraining the patient and these is also the possibility of quite an amount of blood loss from the severed horn stump.

To disbud a calf it is only necessary to wait until it is a few weeks old, as by then the horn bud should be apparent, just coming through the skin. Local anaesthetic is infiltrated around the cornual nerve which runs in a groove between the horn and the corner of the eye. This nerve block works well, and when the hot iron is applied to remove the bud the calf is usually fairly unconcerned. It is best when dealing with goats to dehorn them as early as three days old. To delay any longer than this will mean an increased possibility of the horns regrowing. The common practice, up until a few years ago, was to treat kids like calves and disbud them after local anaesthetic only. This was cruel as even after the best of nerve blocks the young kids would still cry and struggle. For some time now I have made a point of giving all young goats a general anaesthetic. This can be done in a variety of ways but I favour giving them halothane via an oxygen mask. They go to sleep very quickly and are on their feet ready to go home just a few minutes after the operation is finished, seemingly none the worse for the experience.

Most mulilations to animals cannot be condoned and thankfully, in an enlightened society such as ours, those that are still current are losing favour. However, there are still a few which carry on, often to the benefit of the animals concerned, but I do hope that in the future, with better management and understanding, even the need to dehorn, perhaps by only breeding from naturally polled animals, will disappear.

LET US EAT AND DRINK FOR TOMORROW WE DIE

That proverb could have been written for all the animals that we kill and eat for meat. Fortunately the cattle, pigs and sheep in this position have no idea of the fate that awaits them, even as they enter the slaughter house. Their whole existence is concentrated on their need to eat, a biological necessity. The art and science of successful farming is based on feeding farm animals as well and as economically as possible, whether they are for the table or breeding. Livestock farming in the Fens has been on the decline for years, despite the presence of much waste vegetable material which could be utilised for feeding. A very common food still used extensively in this area for fattening cattle is potatoes. It is good and cheap, using only those that are unfit for human consumption, and steers and heifers alike all seem to enjoy eating them raw. All would be well if the diners would only bear in mind "who hastens a glutton, chokes him".

Occasionally, in its haste to consume more than its neighbour, a beast, without chewing properly, will attempt to swallow a tuber that is just too big for its gullet. When this happens, the animal's life is at once put at risk. The clinical picture is alarming, the distracted beast coughs and gags, drooling vast amounts of saliva which it now cannot swallow due to the obstruction. The animal's belly begins to swell up quickly with gas as the blockage prevents its release. Under normal circumstances, this gas which is produced as part of the digestive process of the bovine, is belched up every few minutes. If these vapours are not released within a fairly short period of time, then the beast will die in great distress from circulatory and heart failure.

It's probably still the most common emergency job during the winter months, when the farmers are feeding potatoes or similar materials, like carrots or parsnips. The usual call across the radio is, "Can you go to Mr Crowson's as soon as possible, they have a bullock choking on a potato." On arriving at the scene, if I am lucky, Mr Crowson will have the patient restrained within a cattle crush. If not, the first job is to get it behind a gate where it might be possible to hold and examine it.

Firstly, it is necessary to assess where the obstruction might be. If it's not too far down the neck, it may just be possible to put a hand and arm down the beast's throat, grasp the object and pull it out. It sounds easy, but believe me it's not. Even with the gag in the animal's mouth to stop the back teeth grinding your arm, it feels as if you are being dragged into a mincing machine! My last encounter of this kind left my right arm feeling and looking like a long, raw sausage.

If the obstructing potato is further down the neck, or even within the chest, the proper line of treatment is to push it down the gullet further, and into the stomach by means of an instrument called a probang. This is a semi-rigid tube with a rod down the centre. Up until a few years ago this tube was leather encased with a cane centre rod; these days, as you might imagine, it's made of plastic.

The beast's head is held by the left hand and arm, (to do this it helps if you are built like Geoff Capes), then the right hand passes the instrument down the throat until it touches the blockage. Pressure is then applied by the inner rod of the probang, and in fifty per cent of cases the obstruction is moved down into the stomach, where it is easily digested, and the stomach gas is safely released to the outside world. This gas stinks most dreadfully, and having been within it's range on many occasions has made me much more tolerant of human halitosis.

There are times, however, when nothing will shift the vegetable and it is still imperative to let the gas out as quickly as possible, before the steer dies. Now is the time for a trocar and cannula. This is a fiendish looking piece of equipment, shaped like a dagger. It is inserted through the left flank of the abdomen after a skin incision has been made under local anaesthetic. When it is fully pushed into the animal's stomach or rumen, the trocar is withdrawn, leaving the cannula in position through which the gas escapes. The relief when this is done is very great, to all concerned, particularly the patient. The transformation from dying to near normality within a few seconds is startling. The gas which escapes is mostly methane, and I have often been tempted in the euphoria of the moment to put a light to the gas as it escapes for pyrothenic effect. I believe a German vet did this once, and the flames set fire to a barn and burnt it and its contents to the ground! What happened to the patient was not recorded, but I do know that the vet was sued successfully for a large sum of money.

Having let the gas out of the stomach and made the animal safe, you must not forget the potato is still there blocking the throat. Fortunately, Mother Nature usually comes to the rescue. After a matter of 12-24 hours, the saliva from the mouth causes partial digestion of whatever the vegetable is and softens it. It is then either swallowed or pushed down with the probang, when it is then safe to remove the cannula from the steer's side.

Not all bloat cases are the result of obstruction of the gullet. There can be many different reasons, but one of the commonest is frothy bloat. Gas is suspended in stomach liquid to form a froth which can be just as serious to the beast concerned. This is often the result of over eating; lush, succulent grass can be the worst culprit for causing this problem. When a stomach tube is passed into the rumen and no gas is released, the case is more or less proven to be one of frothy bloat.

Treatment consists of drenching the patient, usually with vegetable oils or silicon compounds, to break up the froth into gas and liquid, and the gas is then expelled in the time honoured manner. There are many times when unfortunately the cause of the bloat remains unknown. However, it can usually be successfully treated whatever the cause if caught in time, but if it recurs frequently and perhaps in the middle of the night the affliction can often prove fatal. When an animal has bloated more than two to three times for no diagnosable reason, then I am often asked by the farmer to operate and make a permanent fistual in the steer's side. This means there is a permanent hole into the animal's stomach through which the stomach gases escape freely all the time.

It is a fairly simple operation which is done under local anaesthetic. A skin incision is made about four to six inches long in the left flank: fingers are then used to break down the muscle fibres all the way to the stomach wall. A pouch of the stomach is then pulled to the exterior, an incision made in it about the same length as the skin cut, and the incised edges of the stomach are then sutured to the skin edges. The hole formed is a permanent one, and the bloat problem is thus instantly overcome. I'm sometimes sorry that God in his wisdom hadn't made all beasts like that, it would certainly have saved a lot of animals lives, and saved the farmers a lot of money!

Cattle that have had the operation usually thrive very well after as they never feel full, and often continue to feed long after their companions have had enough. The only drawback to the procedure is that you have to be very careful how you approach such a beast as you are liable to get covered in stomach contents if it coughs and you are anywhere within range, as the gastric contents can shoot out at an alarming velocity giving you little chance of taking avoiding action!

Never under-estimate bullocks' capacity to eat until they make themselves ill; nor do they necessarily get bloat for their troubles. Often the only consequence is little more than diarrhoea for a day or two which seems to inconvenience them just a little. It may well upset the stockman more if he gets a "shitty" wet tail swished in his face a few times!

There are times though, when cattle over eat the wrong things such as barley meal and they become intoxicated. The cereal ferments inside them causing an acidosis which in the milder cases results in a little drunken stupor: severe cases can die. Treatment consists of intra venous fluids to counter the dehydration and B vitamins to detoxify the system. The braver vets among us have been known to operate, again through the flank, to empty the stomach of it's poisonous contents. If you are not very careful, gastric contents can spill into the abdomen and the patient can end up with a peritonitis as well - and just as dead.

Bovines have been, and still are, fed successfully on all manner of materials including bananas, which to my knowledge one dairy farmer fed to his milking cows! I don't know whether the milk was similarly flavoured, but I do know that he couldn't have fed onions. Another client who did just this swore that his bullocks' breaths tainted everything for hundreds of yards of the cattle shed!

Most animals, whether horses or cattle are curious creatures and will often attempt to eat particularly unsuitable foodstuffs which cause them nothing but harm. There are some poisonous plants they will avoid, like ragwort, unless they are very hungry but there are few animals, given the chance to snatch a piece of yew tree or hedge who will not take it. If they do, it is the last thing they do, as yew is a deadly poison and within minutes of eating it the animal will be dead, as there is no known antidote.

Sheep as a species are not noted for being greedy, but still do suffer like cattle from bloat on occasions. This is usually the frothy type and is normally treated in a like manner to the bovine complaint with oily drenches, but sometimes in an emergency a trocar and cannula has to be used. Those of you who have seen the film from the book "Far From the Madding Crowd" will remember very clearly Gabriel Oak coming to the rescue of Bathsheba's sheep with a trocar after they had got into a field of succulent kale and gorged themselves. Gabriel's histrionic use of the trocar, despite its dramatic effect, is not the recommended method for its use where a little less force and more skill is the order of the day.

Cattle are not the only herbivores to have problems with overeating, gulping their food and choking. Horses, and in particular ponies not infrequently get choked. They rarely, if ever choke on potatoes as they are not fed them as a normal practice. However, especially in the Fens, they do eat carrots which can cause the odd problem but the likeliest cause is dry foodstuffs such as sugar beet pulp or bran; such feed should be thoroughly soaked before use. A pony or horse eating dry food rapidly may get a plug of dry food in the gullet which can create quite an impaction. The animal looks very distressed with its head and neck stretched right out, coughing and with salivary fluids pouring from the nose and mouth. Fortunately it is not a deadly type of emergency as it is in cattle, despite what the owner might think. This is because of the very different type of digestive system compared to cattle, as the horse's organ of digestion is the large intestine and any gas that accumulates in the gut is expelled out the rear end. The usual line of treatment for a choked equine is to give it an antispasmodic drug or sedative, which relaxes the muscles in the throat thus enabling the object to be swallowed. There are times when this is not enough and a stomach tube has to be passed via the nostril and an attempt made to clear the blockage by siphoning out the plug of food. This is a procedure that most ponies don't appreciate, particularly if it has to be repeated a few times, and quite often concludes with everyone getting fed up and the patient's nose bleeding due to the tube irritating the sensitive lining of the nose.

For all this, even with the record for an obstruction lasting for three days, I have yet to loss a horse or pony and they certainly don't get bloated like cattle.

In any mixed practice much time is spent with clients whose pets are seriously overweight. This is the inevitable result of being allowed to eat too much in relation to the amount of exercise that the animal takes. Many practices make a regular income by selling diet food to owners of obese pets who have endangered their animal's health. Diet clinics will soon be a regular part of my practice where dogs and cats will come frequently to be weighed and checked to ensure they are losing the correct amount of weight. It's not uncommon to find at times that the owner or one of the family is cheating by allowing titbits and defeating the whole point of the exercise!

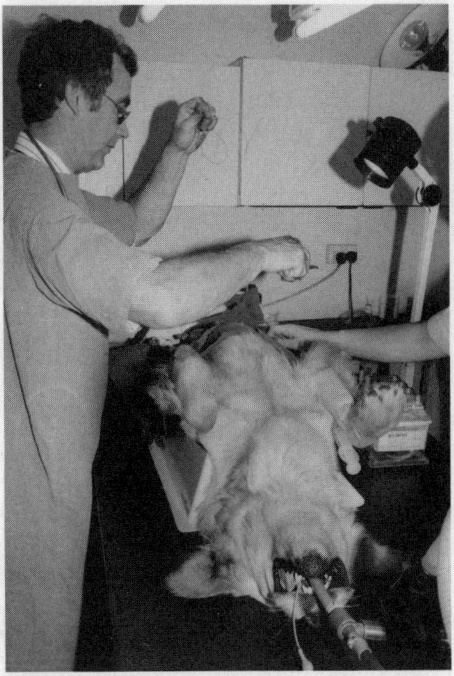

Anna Oakford

The Author stitches up a patient after surgery.

Dogs are particularly renowned for eating all manner of unsuitable items. It's just as well their vomiting mechanism is well developed, as it enables the average canine to get rid of a noxious substance before it does too much harm. Mind you, what we would consider to be fairly revolting, the average pooch often finds quite delectable. I have yet to find a dog that doesn't find horse or cow dung very palatable, and they don't tend to sick it up again either! Perhaps the manufacturers of dog food would be on to a sure fire winner if they marketed a food that tastes of manure; maybe they do for all we know, as I shouldn't think many of us have tasted either to compare!

For all their ease of being sick, there are times when a dog will swallow something very unsuitable and it stays down and results in the animal becoming very ill. These substances could be poisons like chemical sprays or rat poison, either ingested directly or obtained second hand by eating an animal like a rat that has taken the poison in the first instance. Warfarin is a common rat poison which is an anticoagulant. This means that the blood in the victim will not clot and the animal bleeds to death, usually internally. Clinically the dog with Warfarin poisoning is often presented as being cold and clammy to touch, very sleepy with signs of anaemia. It's just as well there is an antidote to this poison and this is vitamin K. This, if injected intravenously, will usually effect a good response providing the patient is not too far gone. Blood transfusions may be necessary in extreme cases.

Many dogs will play with and eat things which even they must know are not food. I have taken all sorts of strange objects out of canine stomachs over the course of the years, and little would surprise me in that department. Needles and hooks are commonly swallowed, and their path through the intestine can be followed until they are normally eliminated at the other end.

It can be difficult diagnostically, if a foreign body is suspected and nothing shows on X ray. Rubber and plastic will not be detected readily on an X ray film, and very often a barium meal has to be given before detection is possible. Even then the picture may not be clear, and in some cases where strong suspicions are aroused that all is not well in the abdomen, an exploratory operation has to be performed.

Many times, however, the owner will present a patient with details of what exactly has been ingested. Labradors are often the worst culprits for eating silly things: one last year was presented as the owner said it had swallowed a mouse. Not much to worry about there, I thought, providing the mouse hadn't been poisoned, all would be well in due course. This was greeted with some doubt by the owner, as the mouse was a large plastic toy one!

On opening the dog's stomach, a large head of a Mickey Mouse look alike appeared, which winked at me with one eye and smiled beguilingly. It also had a most rude note on its nether regions which the embarrassed owner was most anxious to reclaim!

Another Labrador of my acquaintance was very fond of pinching ladies underwear off washing lines, and would not confine his activities to his own garden. This little fetish did not endear him to the neighbourhood. All sorts of maniacs were thought to be on the loose until Sam was discovered to be the culprit.

One Saturday he went too far and swallowed what he chewed, and very rapidly became ill with unproductive vomiting. I spend most of the evening disengaging a pair of ladies tights which had become thoroughly entangled in his small intestine. The operation was difficult and prolonged and Sam was lucky to survive, but I eventually went home quite pleased with my efforts only to discover the next morning that he had done a better job overnight, and brought up the knickers that I hadn't noticed in his stomach!

He survived that time but I heard later when he had moved away from my jurisdiction that he was quite incorrigible, and had died after a similar episode.

Cats are nothing like as troublesome as dogs for swallowing the wrong things, being much more fastidious. It does happen sometimes though and I did have one patient, a Siamese, which after attacking a balloon, ate the knotted end of it. At least that was the owner's explanation. It looked more like remnant of a used condom to me!

It's strange quirk of nature which the uninitiated will find hard to believe, but dogs suffer much like cattle, from bloat. The causes are a little different, and the illness can be even more difficult to treat with the final outcome being much more uncertain. The condition generally only occurs in the giant breeds of dog like the Great Dane or Briard. The dogs usually become bloated after a heavy meal when the stomach rotates either clockwise or anti clockwise producing a functional blockage of the gullet. The stomach and intestines rapidly fill with gas and the dog becomes acutely ill. If the distention is not relieved very quickly the animal dies within a very short period of time. An emergency operation is called for if a stomach tube won't move into the stomach. There may not even be time to scrub up properly or prepare the patient beyond giving it an anaesthetic. Even if the operation is successful in clearing the rotation caused blockage, the patient may still die of toxemia or peritonitis.

After the acute crisis is over, an attempt is often made to anchor the stomach wall to the inner wall of the abdomen, as a recurrence is almost inevitable if you don't.

Gastric torsion and bloat is one more complaint which can be avoided by careful management. Large dogs, despite all folk lore to the contrary, are better fed two or three times a day and should not be allowed exercise until their meal has been digested. That seems simple enough, but this advice seems to be a familiar adage from mother to children, and how much attention did we pay to it then?

CATS AND MOIRA THE CAT LADY

Cats have lived with and among people for many thousands of years, and in that time they have changed very little, being thoroughly self-possessed and independent.

In some cultures, notably in Egypt, they were regarded as Gods and worshipped. At other times they were merely tolerated by societies who only found them useful for keeping vermin at bay. In more recent times, cats were looked on with fear and suspicion as they were thought to be associated with sorcery and witchcraft.

Now, in Britain, cats are more popular than ever before, and there are thought to be about seven million kept as household pets — more than dogs!

The reasons for this are not hard to find. In a society which requires both men and women to go out to work, a cat fits in much more readily being so much more self sufficient than a dog. The majority require only a cat flap and feeding twice daily to remain loyal and happy with a family.

Feral cats are found in many different places and often exist quite happily in an environment which may be considered totally unsuitable by interfering humans. I often feel that these animals would be happier if they were left to their own devices instead of being rescued and neutered.

Unfortunately, feral cats in a semi urban and urban environment, or even on a farm will often breed prodigiously until health problems ensue and something has to be done. If left undisturbed and free of any influence from man, for instance on an island, the cats would maintain themselves at a successful level.

However, given that a colony is getting out of control due to feeding by people and subsequent over breeding, then some rescue societies like the Cats Protection League will trap and neuter the wild cats. When they have recovered from their operation many will then be returned to the colony. This can upset the whole hierarchical set up in the colony as neutered toms lose their status and position in the group. Some, in fact too many, can't be returned and either have to be put down if unwell, or if at all possible found homes on suitable farms where they earn their keep killing vermin.

Cat rescue societies are almost invariably run by women and they are a dedicated band of people. While the majority of women who care and look after cats keep everything within a reasonable perspective, there are a few, and they are usually unmarried ladies, for whom looking after cats becomes a life consuming passion and an obsession. I have known quite a few over the years, dedicated people every one, but one in particular has stood out in that time.

She was called Moira and she came into my part of West Norfolk about fifteen years ago. She was a single woman, an only child whose parents had moved in the very best society circles in London. Indeed I believe her father had been a Lord Lieutenant in one of the Shire Counties somewhere, and needless to say they had been quite well off.

She had been denied the opportunity of marriage, firstly by her parents and then by the death of her fiance during the war. She nursed her parents in their declining years and after they had died she decided from that time on to devote the rest of her life to rescuing and looking after cats.

She moved up to Norfolk like many others before her, due to the attraction of relatively cheap housing, as she now had a limited income. She brought with her from London, along with a few pieces of antique furniture and family silver, about 80 cats and moved into a charming little cottage about a ten minute walk from the nearest village.

Moira was by this time, a fairly elderly lady. Tall and slim, she had a personal charm which did not conceal an inner strength and resolve. You could tell it was not without reason that she was known as the "Duchess" in certain parts of London.

It was shortly after her arrival that I came to know her through a mutual friend. She phoned me and asked if I would be veterinary surgeon to her cats. Initially all was well: together we worked out a programme for neutering and vaccinating all her waifs and strays. Her cats were obviously well looked after and well fed (perhaps better than their keeper), and were housed for the most part in a large shed next to the cottage.

After a few months it became apparent that Moira was losing control of the situation and her charges. They were taking over. The cottage became increasingly over-run with cats; wherever you turned there were cats. When you opened a kitchen cupboard two or three heads would pop out inquiringly. Turn around and pull open a drawer, the same would happen. There would even be cats in the cooker oven — just as well it was never used!

Very soon the house began to look and smell awful. The carpets which had so recently been fitted as new throughout, became sticky to walk on, and you had to be very careful where you sat! The initial programme for neutering and vaccinating had to stop, as Moira's by now meagre income was swamped by the demands of feeding her charges, who increased in numbers almost daily as more cats and kittens were dumped on her. She was known as "The Cat Lady" who never turned away a cat. Inevitably, with so many animals living together many developed health problems, and some died or had to be put to sleep as they became terminally ill.

Moira would never allow any of her dead charges to be taken away, and the dead animal would lie in state in her bedroom for up to a week before she would have them buried in the garden. She did this as she said she wanted to be absolutely sure they were dead before they were buried! As you can imagine, this practice enhanced the smell of the cottage more than somewhat, especially in the summer months!

After about eighteen months, in which time the cottage became more of a health hazard to woman and animals, most of Moira's money had disappeared due to the enormous cost of looking after all her dependents.

She was forced by the bank to sell the cottage, for a lot less than she had paid for it due to its now dilapidated state, and settled into two caravans at the bottom of the garden. One caravan was for Moira to live in and the other, with a large run attached was for the cats.

All too soon the same scenario was reenacted. Cats began to take over her living accommodation again, and the conditions in which Moira had to live became very squalid. To see such a fine old lady destroyed by her love of cats was very sad. She would pay no heed to pleas from friends, relatives or myself that she would have to change her ways and stop the cats over-running her life. She would laugh a little but deny them nothing, and not turn one away. She hardly ate at all while the cats got fatter and more demanding.

Her living caravan became the sort of place you put wellington boots on before you went inside, and just when I and everyone else was about to despair, a little miracle happened.

It was just before Christmas, a new caravan appeared on the scene, financed by some of her relatives. Its facilities were plumbed in and Moira promised all who loved her, especially the nephew who had arranged it all, that she would admit no furry four legged friends within its walls.

That Christmas was for once, clean, dry and warm. Unfortunately by the New Year her resolve had given way. To begin with it was only one or two that "needed special attention", however, the familiar saga had begun again.

All her possessions were being sold off in dribs and drabs to pay the costs of her animals upkeep, and she became so desperate for money she persuaded a local farmer to allow her to work in a gang, cleaning and bagging carrots and parsnips. It was payment by results, and inevitably because her by now emaciated body tired readily and her fingers were crippled with arthritis, very little was earned.

Many people tried to help, but any food that was given for her own consumption was consumed by her cats, and I think she existed on very little at all. Efforts to persuade her that the cats would have to go or she would die looking after them were met with a smile, which although never stated, meant that she knew no finer fate.

She nearly got her wish when she collapsed, exhausted, and was taken off to hospital. No one could take care of her charges and it was decided, quite rightly, by the local authority that the R.S.P.C.A. would have to sort the mess out.

A very understanding inspector took charge, and large numbers of semi wild cats were trapped, some were re-homed but the majority had to be put down.

When Moira came out of hospital, her caravan having been condemned, she was found a home in a local authority cottage to which she retired with her three remaining cats. She settled down, and with the help of friends the house soon became cosy and comfortable, and no more cats were allowed to be dumped on her.

Old habits die hard however, and a stray Collie she called Kim, who had lived rough on the estate soon made his home with her. They became devoted to each other, and the cats accepted him as one of the family.

She settled into a more comfortable old age, but her concern for the welfare of animals continued. She would write and telephone statesmen and church leaders on the subject of any current animal cruelty case. The Pope and Archbishop of Canterbury were on her mailing list. She became very cross about one particular Bishop who not only would not listen to her, but actually put the phone down on her. "Not very Christian" she said.

As she now had only a few animals, I didn't see her so often but I continued to pop in if I was in her locality. One of her cats called Susie, whom she always affirmed was female, was one of the biggest, brawniest tom cats I have ever had to treat! Moira could never understand why Susie felt obliged to go out regularly and patrol the neighbourhood. He/she would often come back with a bit missing and an abscess forming from yet another fight. Moira in the end understood, only after I told her that any self respecting tom cat would have to fight when it was called Susie, if only to live down the shame of its name!

On one occasion I was called to see Susie, after yet another night out, and on my arrival he disappeared in the bedroom. It's not uncommon to have to search a lady's bedroom for a patient, and I was on my hands and knees beside the bed, peering under it. Without

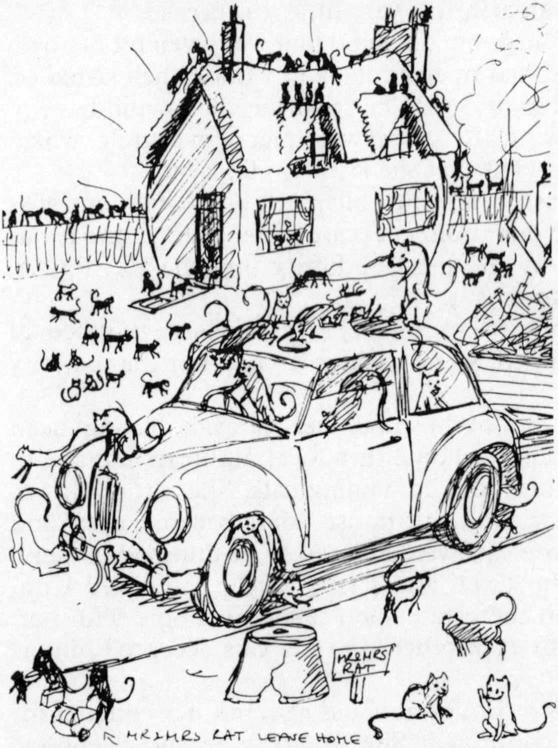

thinking, I pulled a cord which I thought activated a light. A few moments later, the disembowelled voice of the complex warden came from the corner of the room.

"Are you all right Miss M....?"

"Oh yes" came the reply "I'm just under the bed with my vet."

I learned to be more careful after that!

Moira only had a comparatively short time in her new home before she had another fall and became more debilitated, no doubt brought on by the appalling living conditions she had endured. By now she was very practical, and had a local undertaker visit her to make all the necessary arrangements for her funeral. She was positively gleeful when she told me what she had done. I, for my part, had to promise to put her three cats to sleep after her death, as she rightly realised that to re-home her old friends would not only be almost impossible, it would also be unkind. Kim, I assured her, would be found the very best of homes.

Not long after these arrangements were made, Moira died, and after the funeral I returned to the cottage for the last time to carry out my promise to her.

Two of the cats were easily found and peacefully put down, but I could not find Susie anywhere. My nurse and I searched high and low without result, until I remembered the old caravan and cottage days and pulled out a drawer in the bedside cabinet. Sure enough, there he was, in a very comfortable bolt hole. It was a very bleak ending in that by now, very cold little house, but I had carried out the dying wishes of an old friend, who with the very best of motives had died as she had lived, putting the care and welfare of her animal friends before any personal considerations.

TO EVERY MAN (ANIMAL) . . .

Many people believe that one of the most important services that a veterinary surgeon can give his patients when the time is right, is euthanasia. To relieve an animal's suffering when there is no hope of a cure, has to be one of the most important duties a vet can have. Yet I find it is a responsibility which weighs ever more heavy as I get older. I suppose it's like the old adage, the more you see the less you know, or the more animal lives you have to end the harder it gets. Perhaps it's just as well; if it got easier then I suspect I would on occasions, be failing in my care for my patients. If often feels, as I make my way around the Fen, that I am dealing out drugs with one hand (in the form of licensed medicines in case I excite the unwarranted attentions of the constabulary), and death with the other.

At the beginning of my veterinary career, whilst a working student, I had a robust, no-nonsense attitude to killing an animal. It came from having a farming background. Life and death were very much part of the environment and treated in a natural, matter of fact manner. I was first made aware that not everyone shared my lack of sensibilities when I was "seeing practice" as a student. I was with a vet doing his morning rounds and had been called to a house to attend a sick dog. This had been duly and satisfactorily sorted out when en route to the car through the garden the dog's owner noticed an injured bird on the pathway. He picked it up and asked me to look at it. A moments glance told me it would never fly again and I quickly, and somewhat expertly for me, broke its neck and put it out of its misery; whereupon I was taken to task very thoroughly by the dog's owner who had expected me to carry it off and "take care of it properly". The vet, in private, later told me I had done the right thing but at the wrong time as I had not considered the client's feelings.

This need to be more aware of the client's finer feelings was reinforced some weeks later when I had to accompany another veterinary surgeon to an old lady's house to see a sick budgie. As ill-fortune would have it, the bird had an inoperable tumour and had to be put down. The lady was heart broken as this little animal was the only company she had had since her husband died. She loved it and was going to miss it dreadfully. It was a very bare room in a small house, lacking most of the usual amenities, and it was made to feel all the more bleak by her tears. We took every care to comfort her before we removed the budgie and humanely destroyed it with chloroform. We wrote to her afterwards and explained again why her pet had to die and were rewarded with a charming letter in return, thanking us for our care. That one case taught me more about how to handle grief and how to be more aware of people's feelings when a pet has to be put down than any number of lectures.

For many people, their dog, car or other pet (not to be too specific), is to them a faithful companion, a member of the family and often a child substitute. When it has to be put down, the owner will often feel a mixture of emotions from grief to anger and often guilt. The oft repeated question is "would it have made any difference if I had called you in sooner?" Sometimes the honest answer would be "yes", but it is often not said, as that usually doesn't serve any useful purpose, unless another animal is at risk.

It is often very difficult to gauge how different people will react to their animals dying. Seeming indifference and outwardly callous, joking demeanour can often be a mask to hide deep distress. Not long after the Falklands campaign, a soldier came to me with his old dog. It was at least eighteen years old, its teeth were rotten, it was crippled with arthritis and could hardly walk, despite being very thin. It was in terminal kidney failure, and it was going to be kinder by far to put it to sleep than subject it to hospitalisation and treatment. Drips and medicines at best could only give a few more, possibly pain filled weeks. Given this choice the soldier made the sensible decision to put an end to his dog's suffering. This conclusion was reached in a brusque, off hand manner, but when he came to hold the dog for the injection, he broke down completely and wept. He said later that he had been in the thick of the conflict at Goose Green and had seen both friends and enemies die, but that had not touched him so hard as holding his own dog as it died.

For me personally, I find it much more difficult as a man, to cope with another man in tears. The male is brought up with the ethos than it is unmanly to weep, and when he does he is often embarrassed as well as distressed for his pet. Women cry more readily, without shame, and I know that this release of emotion is essential to help them over the mourning period. Mourning a much loved pet is as normal and necessary as grieving for a human, and it's a pity that so many are often ashamed to admit it.

I suppose that most people believe that the vet's job is done when the syringe is empty and the animal is dead, but I find this very far from being the case. Apart from writing a letter, mostly to assure the owner that their decision has been the correct one for their pet, and that to have delayed any longer would have increased the animal's suffering, we are also within the practice involved with funeral arrangements. Many owners wish to have their animals cremated and their ashes returned, and this we can, and do organise. There was a time not so long ago, when it was not so unusual for an owner to want to have their dear departed stuffed, and I always had the phone number of the local taxidermist to hand. Fortunately this trend seems to have ebbed somewhat of late. Others have asked undertakers to make proper coffins and to attend to the arrangements for them. Indeed, there are now companies who will organise coffins and burials for any pet, large or small, from a cat to a horse. A client of some years ago always made his own dog's coffins in oak. They were very robust structures and they needed to be, as when he moved house, which was at least twice while I knew him, the coffins were exhumed and put in the removal van to be reburied in the new garden!

My most enduring memory of a dog's funeral was for a gun dog owned by a close friend. Old Bob had served my friend well over many years, and when he had to be put down he was buried with full shooting honours under the chestnut tree in the back garden. I was invited to attend, and was asked to fire a shot over his grave as a parting salute. This, with all due solemnity was what I did and was nudged by my friend to do the job properly by firing the second barrel. We then retired to the front parlour to drink a toast to his memory.

What I have recounted so far has been mostly about small animals, but I have to confess that the hardest job of all is to put down a horse or pony. It really, rationally, should not be the case. Horses or ponies are euthanased (horrible word) by me, only if they are in pain which cannot be relieved, such as is caused by a shattered limb or a twisted bowel. Only occasionally is it because the animal is old and completely worn out.

Whatever the reason, and however correct the decision, when it comes to putting the gun to the forehead, between the brown, trusting eyes and pulling the trigger, I have yet to feel anything but regret, remorse and sick at the violent end to the animal's life.

As you might expect, however, even with death as a subject, there are some lighter moments. We do have our share of eccentric clients, and very few compare with one gentleman who shuffled through our doorway some years ago. He was a man of perhaps some sixty years with a somewhat dishevelled appearance, a belligerent expression, and a loud voice. He came up to the reception desk and I could tell from his manner that he was going to give the nurse a difficult time. Anticipating this I intercepted him,, and asked if I could help.

"Yes" came the reply "I want my dog done in."

Now we never agree to that sort of request without finding out first what the problem is. I took him to the nearby consulting room to question him further, as it is often possible to re-home an unwanted pet. Safely within the privacy of the room I asked "What's the matter with the dog?"

"Well master" he said prodding me in the chest with his fore finger "It's not the dog, it's the vacuum cleaner that's the problem. My old hoover has broken down, I've got to get a new one but it's no good, the dog has got to go." I had some difficulty making the connection between cleaner and dog, but he soon explained in his own inimitable manner.

It seemed that until it broke down, his old cleaner would pick up the dog dirt in the house (that was not quite his choice of words, I have altered a few so as not to offend too many sensitive feelings - which is something my client clearly didn't consider!). He had tried to get the old machine repaired, but to no avail as the repair man wouldn't touch it. He had bought a new cleaner and tried that, but it was no good, it couldn't pick up like the old one. He even complained to the shop where he had bought it but there was nothing else they could do, and "NO" they would not refund his money!

Faced with an obviously incontinent dog whose re-homing prospects were nil, it was obvious that the old thing would have to go. I agreed to his proposition and gave him an appointment for that afternoon.

"No, no mate" came the reply "I can't do that yet, I've only just bought a new load of dog food, and its got to eat that first!" With that, he went off down the drive still muttering and complaining about British workmanship and new cleaners. I wasn't too surprised or disappointed that he and his dog failed to keep the appointment made for the following week, and I never saw him again!

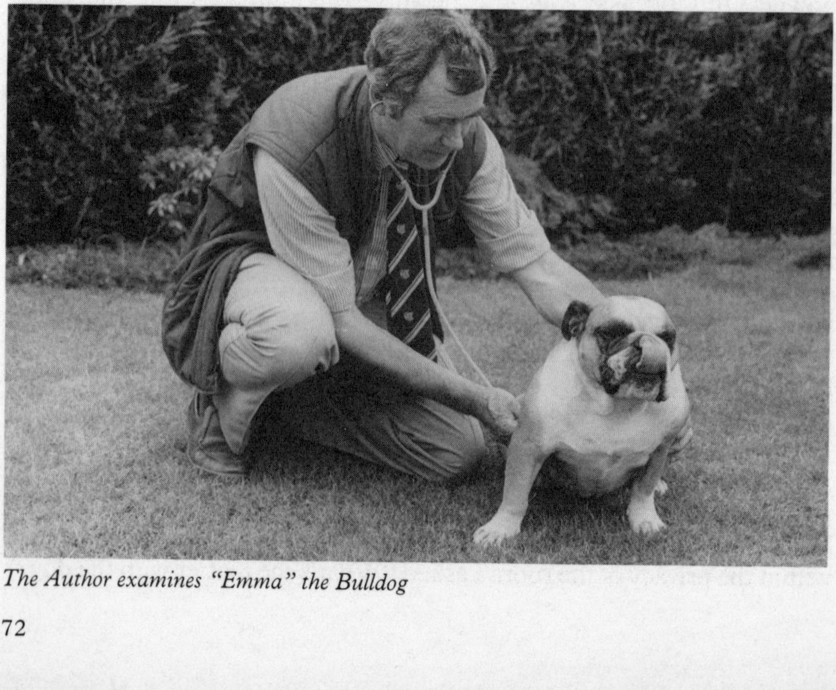

Anna Oakford

The Author examines "Emma" the Bulldog

AS SICK AS A PARROT

It would be great to be given fifty pence (I'm taking account of inflation)!, for every time a patient's owner said to the vet "you must be more clever than a doctor as your patient can't tell you where the pain is".

Now I would be the last one to deny such a premise, but the idea that those that we look after can't communicate is entirely a false one. The odd thing is, that those animals who have the ability to talk can actually communicate less than most dogs, despite Esther Rantzen trying to prove otherwise!

The average parrot is dirty, devious, and despite any degree of loquacity on its part, is totally uncommunicative on why it might be feeling ill or where the pain might be.

My first ever encounter with such a pet (or did I mean pest)? happened on a night of freezing fog. I had to travel a round trip of twenty four miles to see a bird whose owner thought it was extremely ill. It was ill, mentally ill, a neurotic wreck! Completely bald from the neck down, it was spending its time scampering around the cage like an over active John Cleese. At the first sign of a feather emerging from one of its skin follicles, it would emit a screech of demented pleasure and pluck it out!

Polly was very uninformative as to why it was so doing, but after a fairly cursory examination of the skin I didn't think the problem was a physical one. I think most of you would probably have felt the same as it did, given a small cage with nothing to do. I decided the cure might be a matter of giving some other type of recreation and some parrot company. It went back to the pet shop from which it was purchased, and I believe made a quick and uneventful recovery.

Budgies, as you may have noted elsewhere, are one of my favourite small animals. Their ability to chatter away quite intelligibly to their owners, and keep themselves amused is a delight to behold, but they might just as well be talking in Swahili as far as I am concerned as I can never understand a word. Usually the proud owner has to stand and translate every utterance before I get the gist of what they are saying, and it's not usually worth waiting for when it comes. If you are waiting for a list of symptoms from it, forget it! However, you might just get some help from the owner.

Some years ago now, I was called to an old lady's house in Chatteris to see her budgie who was reported as being very sick. The bird was huddled in a corner of her cage, her feathers were fluffed up and she had been vomiting.

A clinical examination of the bird failed to show the cause of the disorder, and I was puzzled, until I asked for a little history, then all was revealed. Most evenings the budgie was in the habit of sitting on her owner's shoulder, chirping in her ear, and accepting a little piece of whatever her owner was eating or drinking. The previous night it happened to be gin and tonic they were sharing. The budgie had had one sip too many and was paying the price of overindulgence with a hangover! The cure was a little extra warmth and a blanket over the cage to cut out the light for a few hours, and she was as good as new in the morning.

So you can forget about getting any help in your diagnosis from a prattling parrot or a bumptious budgie!

Thankfully, from the vet's point of view, most of our patients do communicate in a way which the behavioural experts call "body language". Put at its most basic, this means that if you touch a sore place in a dog, it might turn around and bite you! A cat may scream, claw and bite you, and the larger animals may attempt all three plus kick - all at the same time if you are unlucky. If you are looking at a camel, they spit as well! There are times when you have to be quite fleet of foot to survive.

As veterinary students, many hours are spent examining and trying to understand all the signs that we get from our patients in order to know what is wrong with them. Where difficulties can arise is when we have to deal with something a bit more exotic than the average pet or farm animal.

I see and treat quite a lot of foxes; these are usually obtained as very small cubs, dug out of earths with their mother, and after killing the vixen, no one had the heart to kill the youngsters. I don't like seeing wild animals kept in captivity, as mostly they seem to have a fearfully restricted existence, and rarely to my mind become domesticated.

One exception to this was a fox called "Winky Woo". It too had been obtained as a cub, but its owners had given a great deal of thought, time and money into making it an environment in which it seemed entirely happy. it had a large outside run with lots of toys that it seemed to enjoy, and also through a series of flaps it could come into the house without the risk of escaping. It also used to play with the family dog and cats and appeared to be totally happy and integrated.

All was well for many years, then it seemed to develop toothache symptoms. It wasn't possible to look in its mouth without sedation, and when this was done it was found to have cancer in its mouth. This was treated with excision, and at the owners insistence, Winky

Woo had radiation therapy at a treatment centre in Newmarket. This prevented the cancer from spreading and recurring for some months, but at the end of that time it still had to be put down. I'm not happy to this day that we were justified in putting the creature through that treatment, as I was never sure whether it was concealing the pain and distress signals that I would have picked up from a dog.

Other foxes I have treated, have shown all too clearly the pain of captivity, even those that are captured as cubs. One such case involved a dog and a vixen who were kept together for a number of months, growing together and playing together. The dog was castrated for obvious reasons, but one night a wild fox came along and dug the vixen out of the compound, leaving her castrated mate behind. The dog remained in captivity for about eighteen months after this, visited periodically by the liberated vixen who would invariably call at night time.

He died quite suddenly without showing any physical reason for ailing, and while I hesitate to be emotive about the subject, I think he just lost the will to live. He had looked a very lonely, miserable creature, and everyone who looked at him felt sorry, but to have released him would have been doubly unkind as he couldn't have survived in what to him was a hostile environment. Better by far if he had been killed with his mother than undergo the torture of captivity, and the loss of his litter mate and friend.

Not all wild animals are unhappy about captivity. I still chuckle over a recent incident when a friend phoned me to ask my opinion about an animal he had rescued. He described it as a small furry creature which he had found sitting in the middle of a road. It was very quiet and was easily persuaded into a cage where it was kept for a few days, being fed on all manner of goodies.

James (my friend) had a dawning of suspicion as to the identity of the animal when he brought it to the surgery for identification. It was a large, brown, very common rat. Quite happy in its cage, it was sitting up chewing a delicacy. James was more than a little embarrassed at this revelation and asked what he should do with it. No lover of vermin, I told him what he should do, but I knew from the look on his face that he wouldn't. He had grown quite attached to it having fed and looked after it for a few days.

He took it down a country lane, opened the cage door and let it out, and it scurried off in true rat fashion without so much as a grateful backward glance. It was obviously restored to full health by James's careful nursing. Now if it had been able to communicate, I'm sure it would have been crafty enough to keep quiet about its true identity!

We learn about animals' illness or behaviour, not only from the animals themselves, but also as I've said before, by questioning or taking a history from the owner. Some owners are very good at recounting all the relevant details required, almost too good in some cases, as there are times you get swamped by an owner branding copious notes. Others are hopeless, but it also helps of course, if the communication is a two way process, as it is no good asking questions if you don't listen to the answers! Or if you only hear what fits your provisional diagnosis.

A good example of this happened to me some years ago, and it could have had a very sorry outcome. Two gentlemen bought a very large, fierce German Shepherd dog into the consulting room and asked me to put it to sleep. I didn't question them further but as it was so large and fierce, I decided to give it a sedative injection first, before I attempted to administer the lethal jab.

I did this, and after a time the dog became very sleepy, and as part of the general conversation I asked why they wanted the dog put down. There was immediate consternation at this; they wanted the dog put to sleep so that I could safely look in his ears and treat them for canker - not put to sleep as in euthanasia, kill it! Fortunately for all concerned, including the dog, the sedative was reversible, and as the dog came round it exacted its revenge by biting me.

That taught me a large lesson, not least to listen to people properly, and if there is any doubt about the matter to get the owner to sign a consent form for any procedure you may be about to inflict on their pet! The lesson that you must listen to what the owner is telling you is an obvious one, but you must also learn to draw your own conclusions from the evidence.

I have had many telephone conversations with owners recounting their pet's symptoms, but few more strange than the hysterical lady who commanded my immediate presence at her home, where she was sure her beloved dog was dying. Further questioning revealed that the said pet was at that very moment at the bottom of the garden, digging a hole just as fast as he could. The poor lady would not be convinced other than he was digging his own grave. I had this Monty Python image of a fat little beagle, as such it was, furiously trying to complete his task before he expired! Off course I went straight away. The patient had been off colour for a day or two and was feeling sick. What in fact it was doing, being a very clean little dog, was vomiting in the prepared hole and then covering the evidence.

An anti vomit injection and some antibiotic cured the patient, and a large sherry for the owner and a small one for the vet restored sanity to the household. The dog had been giving all the right signals, it was just the owner that misinterpreted them!

Training any animal to do any task is all about communication. Providing they know quite clearly what you want them to do, and there is a reward at the end of the exercise if they do it well, then most animals, and dogs in particular, will respond with enthusiasm. The same can be said about handling them. If you are firm, strong and dominant, without trying to frighten, then the majority of pets will respond in a positive manner.

Cats, for example, can be very fractious in a consulting room, but if you hold them tightly by the scruff and turn them on their backs, the majority will quieten into calm little pussy cats. Don't attempt to turn a dog on its back in the same way in order to restrain it, it doesn't work, allow them to keep all four feet on the ground or they panic!

Horses too, respond to quiet sympathetic handling, but like children need to know that if they step out of line, retribution awaits them. Be fair, be consistent, be firm and be kind, but not soft. Any animal, be it dog, horse or whatever, knows when you are frightened and will use that knowledge to their advantage.

Many times I've had a dog in the consulting room, ruffled its ears, taken its temperature and conducted a full examination without a hint of trouble: at the end the owner has stood back and said "Well, no one has been able to do that before!" Being unaware of an animal's reputation often gives a confidence to treat it in a matter-of-fact manner to which the dog responds. However, the next time around, the dog knows that you know its reputation and the chances are it will become difficult to handle, because your own inner chemistry will have altered to be ready to cope with any aggression!

Consulting rooms can be very frightening places for patients and owners. Patients because they may associate them with being hurt or just because it's strange to them. Owners can be frightened, worrying about what the vet might say is wrong with their pet, and perhaps about the expense of a possible operation! Vets too can have worrying moments in the surgery, and mostly this is the result of faulty communication.

It's not uncommon to have some clients, who for varying reasons best known to them, like to keep to one particular veterinary surgeon. A middle aged lady came into reception without an animal or an appointment, asked to see me and no one else would do. I was out on a call, but she was determine to wait, and did so. When I came in I took her into the consulting room and asked how I could help her. She burst into floods of tears and told me her daughter was pregnant. Not knowing the lady, I was a little taken aback, and it was some minutes before I had the situation under control.

The essence of the problem was that not only was her sixteen year old daughter pregnant, but so also was her cat, and that was the last straw that had caused all the tears! As it was, all she wanted from me was a promise to operate on her cat as soon as possible, which I did, but I'll admit she had me a bit worried with her first outburst! It's just as well I had a clear conscience at the time.

An even worse experience happened with another lady in the same consulting room, some time after the first incident. She had brought her dog to see me, and at the end of the examination she pressed a letter into my hand telling me I had to open it in private and to let no one see the contents. I thanked her for it, left her in the waiting room and scuttled off to the office to open my envelope expecting a tip (at least a tenner I thought). Instead, the envelope contained a letter, which to my acute embarrassment and consternation turned out to be a proposal of marriage! Much to the amusement of the office staff, to whom I had appealed for help, I hid myself away in the computer room and refused to come out until she had gone away. I certainly didn't want to communicate any more with her, I didn't think my wife would understand. I'm sure the lady didn't really mean the letter for me in particular, I just happened to be there at the right time!

Communication within the practice between vet and lay staff is all important for the efficient running of the business. To this end, we have radio telephones in our cars and personal pagers. These can be a great boon, but also at times a real pain in the neck if you want a quiet half hour to yourself. Needless to say, some of us are more conscientious than others when it comes to answering the devices.

David for example, a vet I used to employ, never seemed to answer the radio telephone at all: you could never get him. He always had an excuse.

"I was out of range", "I was out of the car", or "The dratted machine wasn't working". I had it checked a few times, and it always seemed to be O.K. David was a bit of a hairy driver, and one afternoon hurrying about his business, he took a bend too fast and rolled the car upside down onto a grass verge. He called the surgery for help using the radio whilst hanging upside down in the car, and with the aerial firmly embedded in the mud! Strangely enough, it worked perfectly then, and I never believed any excuses about a faulty radio after that!

You also have to be most careful what you say over the airways. Correct radio procedure should be maintained at all times according to the licensing authorities. None the less, in the heat of the moment, things can be said, which taken out of context can sound a bit strange.

I had occasion to go out to a cow having difficulty calving and suspected the need for a caesarean section and warned the nurses to be on standby. As often happens when you suspect the worst, it doesn't happen and the cow was delivered of her burden without too much difficulty. Somewhat elated, I radioed in to tell all and sundry that it was all right "I have got it out and I'm coming in". I couldn't understand what all the giggling was about, until a kindly soul repeated what I had said.

I seem to have strayed some way from my sick parrot and talking to animals, but it's all about communication, one with the other, and when it breaks down I'm often comforted with the parting words of a professor of medicine at my last external examination before I became a vet.

"Now never forget laddie, vitamin and mineral deficiencies in birds often lead to bare breasts and other vices". Now if he can say silly things out of context and get away with it, then there must still be some hope for me!

THE BITER, BITTEN

Generally speaking, the veterinary profession as professions go is a high risk one. Although, it has to be said, that our average lifespan is on the whole a longer one than those of our medical and dental colleagues. Early on in college life, I was warned to take care with a scalpel as "vets often cut themselves". Once qualified, I repeated this adage to a farmer to be met with a horrified expression. I later learned that the term "to cut" means in this part of the world (the Fens), to castrate, which was not what I had meant at all!

One of the hard facts of life that every aspiring veterinary surgeon has to come to terms with, is that by and large their patients are not in the least grateful for the attention they are receiving. In fact, every now and then a patient will take a violent dislike to them and will do their utmost to bite, kick or maim the vet in any way they can. It's hardly surprising, considering that most animals when they are examined and treated are usually frightened, in pain or both.

Most of the time, a dangerous situation can be anticipated, precautions taken, and all is well. However, exceptions to this rule do occur, and sometimes an animal with predetermined malice, probably as a result of an earlier encounter, will attempt to catch you unprepared.

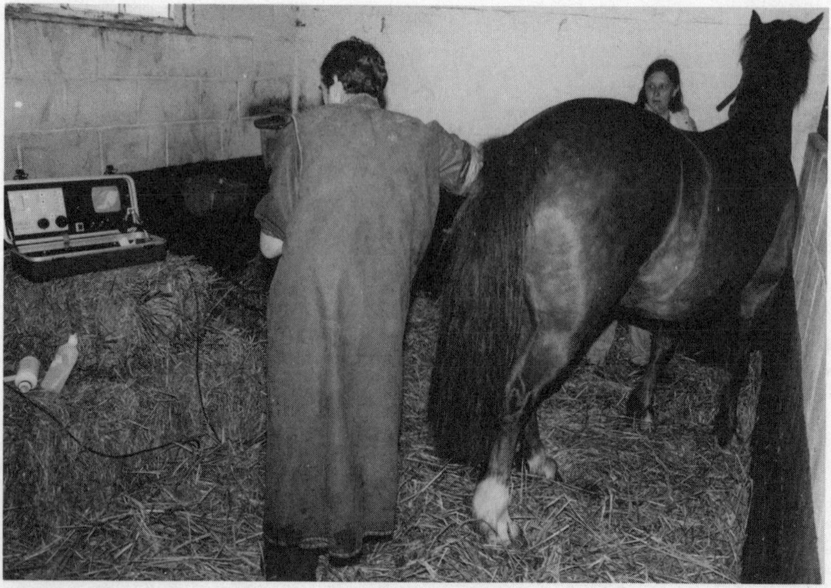

Anna Oakford

Russell Lyon pregnancy scanning a Welsh Section D mare.

Some years ago I was called to a house where the family Labrador was reputed to be in some pain and requiring attention. I knew the family quite well and was received most warmly when I called. The dog was in the back garden, and so accompanied by the husband and wife, out we went to view the patient. I knew from previous meetings with the dog that he was of an uncertain temperament, but I was not expecting too much trouble.

On seeing the deputation, 'Sam', helpful as ever, took himself off to the bottom of the garden and refused all commands to come back. Instead of going to get him and putting him on a lead, the master of the household suggested that Sam might come back if he was bribed with a dish of his absolute favourite, milk. I should have vetoed this immediately, but taking the line of least resistance, agreed to the proposal.

The milk was produced without delay, and sure enough it had the desired effect. Sam duly arrived back to seek his reward. The plan of campaign was, that as soon as he settled to his drink I was to creep up behind him, drop a leash over his head and all would be well.

I approached him from behind and got to within two yards of him, when he turned around and without a moment's hesitation, launched himself straight at my throat! He was a vision of bared yellow fangs, dripping with milk, and hatred filled eyes. He thought, I'm sure, that I was going to take his milk away from him. Self preservation, not having time to run, make me stick out my hands and arms to fend him off, and I found myself catching him in mid flight on his route toward my neck. I was left holding him at arm's length with my hands, fortuitously clasped on either side of his collar. We tumbled over, bowled by the force of his attack and continued our battle on the grass. He, doing his damndest to get me, and I for my part, having lost all sense of dignity, was just trying my best to keep him out of reach of my face and hands!

I looked around, desperate for assistance, only to find that both husband and wife had mysteriously disappeared. After what seemed like an eternity, as the slavering jaws were getting ever closer, we eventually recognised a stalemate, and Sam broke off his attack and disappeared into the shrubbery.

After a few moments to recover and a cup of restorative coffee, I decided to put off the examination for another day. Sam was brought round to the surgery next morning, suitably sedated by some pills I had left for the purpose, and he was no more trouble to deal with. His attack was entirely my own fault as I should have foreseen the likely sequel of events. All that was wrong with him, I discovered, was a bit of arthritis for which there is as yet no cure, but we can at least make the patient's life more comfortable. As it turned out we were both soon swallowing the same type of pain killers, as I was a bit stiff and sore myself after our encounter.

Veterinary surgeons spend a lot of time preaching the virtues of preventative medicine. Prevention is always better than cure, both for the patient and the owner. However, it is still for our "fire brigade role" that the veterinary profession is best known. In an emergency situation, where anything can happen, there is a very fine line between looking quite a competent individual or an absolute fool. It is for this reason, I was told by a colleague while I was working with him as a student, never to show pain if you are hurt by a patient in the course of your duties. It makes you feel twice the fool you might already look. He amply illustrated the point for me not long afterwards, when as a team we were trying to restrain a pain maddened bullock. We had a rope on its head but despite this, we were pulled, with the vet in the lead, through a wooden fence. Apart from a short earthy curse, which was not like him, and looking a bit shaken, he carried on and finished the job., He was a bit quiet for the rest of the day, but didn't seem to restrict or stint himself in any way. I found out some weeks later, that he had actually cracked two ribs as his chest went through the fence. What a man! I'm sure, wimp that I am, that I could never have managed a similar performance.

Of course, any one handling animals is likely to get hurt at some time or another, even the most experienced. But there are other times when you can almost see an accident before it happens. The unwary might step behind a flighty horse and get kicked. The inexperienced might go in with a savage sow with her piglets to protect, and get badly bitten for his trouble. Farmers are usually pretty good at helping a new graduate avoid the pitfalls of being in the wrong place at the wrong time. This is particularly true if the vet in question is young and female. There are times, though, when even the most patient man can be a little exasperated.

A young colleague came back to the surgery one afternoon and recounted standing beside a rather awkward horse while the farmer held it for examination and resultant injection. The horse proved a little difficult and was prancing about. Eventually, the farmer couldn't stand the tension, which was increasing by the minute, and said with some degree of exasperation.

"I shouldn't stand there looking like that if I were you"

"Oh" came the response "and why not?"

"Well if the damned horse doesn't kick you on the arse then I will!"

Farmers themselves are not immune to being hurt either. About two summers ago, on a lovely balmy evening, I was attending to a heifer having calving difficulties She was frightened and difficult, but eventually I got a rope and then a halter on her. The farmer and I attempted to get her to the fence and tied up, when she turned round quite casually and knocked the farmer into the fence. There was quite an audible crack, which I thought was the fence breaking, only to realise a moment later that it was John's right arm that had caused the noise as it had snapped.

He slumped to the ground in considerable pain, and all thoughts for the heifer had to be forgotten for the moment.

It was quite some time before the ambulance came, and I was very tempted to give him some pain killer out of my large animal bag. However, I resisted the temptation, which was just as well as I wasn't too sure of the dose for a person, and I just made him as comfortable as possible with a sling, until professional medical help arrived. By the time we had him packed off to hospital, we were in total darkness and the beast still required attention.

It was just as well for her sake, that on examination I found she wasn't quite ready to give birth. I injected her to delay the onset of second stage labour until it was daylight. I went back to her at 6am, and with the able assistance of my youngest daughter, Kate, delivered with some difficulty, a fine bull calf. I think it was of some consolation to John, lying in his hospital bed, that at least we got a live calf, even if he couldn't be there are the birth.

You might think that dealing with large animals carries more risk to life and limb than caring for pet animals. This, I have to say, has not been my experience, as I've had more bites than kicks in my time. As I have already explained, it is much easier to anticipate when a horse or farm beast is going to have a go at you. I have yet to be bitten by a dog if I have been warned about its temperament. It's always the unexpected that finds you vulnerable: when it does happen there is little you can do about it 'Let the vet beware' is the owner's motto. I have, up until now, resisted the temptation to add a bit on the bill for wear and tear to the nervous system, but I'm not sure I will always hold out. It's not often there is any redress against the patient, but just occasionally a clinical decision will make you feel better!

It was a pretty miserable winter's morning, and I was standing somewhat wearily on the doorstep of a house in Wisbech, having just rung the bell. I was halfway through my opening spiel of "Good morning, how are you, where is the patient?" when this bloody great Alsatian (sorry German Shepherd dog) came hurtling round the corner of the house and grabbed my thigh in an all embracing, teeth clenching (both his and mine) jaw lock! I leapt forward emitting something between a high pitched scream and a falsetto giggle. "My heck", said the lady of the house, as she stood at the door, "The dog's bit the Vet, I told you Dad to hold onto him." Dad had only just arrived, seconds too late to witness the scene of the altercation.

With the ensuing noise and confusion, "Sabre", the cause of all the trouble, took the opportunity to slip away unnoticed, while I did my best to compose myself.

"Are you all right young man?" said Dad, stifling a grin with difficulty, as the world knows there is nothing funnier than the vet getting bitten. It's like one more victory for the under dog. I leant against the door frame and could feel this warm fluid trickling down the back of my leg. "Relax" I thought "It's only blood." I put my hands down the back of my trouser leg, and was relieved to find only the holes where the teeth went in, and no tearing of material. The trousers were more or less intact.

The good lady, showing more concern than dad, offered me the use of the bathroom to further examine the extent of my injuries, but remembering my old mentor, "and never show pain", this was turned down with thanks. Instead, I turned my attention to the patient, who was soon discovered hiding under the kitchen table. The reluctant Sabre was soon dragged out by Dad, and this time suitably restrained and muzzled, was presented for examination. It didn't take too long to discover the cause of the dog's bad temper. He had an all too apparent lump on his bottom, which, without too much doubt was diagnosed as a cancerous growth called an Anal Adenoma. The best treatment for the dog was an operation to remove the mass, and as soon as possible, as it was getting rather large and tended to bleed.

As part of the treatment, as well as excision, most veterinary opinion is that the animal should be castrated at the same time. This is to try and prevent the tumour, which is male hormone dependent, from regrowing once it has been removed.

I thought the matter over for a few minutes, and while I hope it was only clinical considerations which came to mind, my ultimate decision on Sabre's treatment eased the throbbing of my leg considerably!

WHENEVER YOU OBSERVE . . .

"When ever you observe an animal closely, you feel as if a human being inside were making fun of you."

I was kicked on the head by a pony today (my brain does need a kick start now and then), and it made me think of the risks we all run when we look after animals. I was attempting to rasp the animal's teeth as they had some sharp edges, when it reared up and whacked me on the skull with a fore foot. How it achieved this despite being sedated and held quite firmly by its owner, I'm still not quite sure.

On its behalf, I would have to admit that I did have its tongue pulled out to one side to allow me to have a metal instrument in its mouth. The grating noise the rasp makes as it does the job must cause a strange ringing sensation in the head, much worse than the dentist's drill sounds to us. The pony did win the first round by a knock down, and I swear it had a malicious twinkle in its eye as it observed the havoc it had created. I had my way in the end by giving it more sedative, but it yet again emphasised just how dangerous animals can be when they realise how much stronger they are than their human handlers.

I have found, over the years, that most of the time, behavioural problems in animals are mostly the result of poor and sometimes non existent training at an early age. It is a common problem, particularly with foals and yearlings that have not been handled from birth. When eventually you try to restrain them, it is much more traumatic both for the animal and the owner. It is better by far to handle youngsters right from the start, as soon as the maternal bond has been established, and get them used to wearing a headcollar. In this way, training can be an enjoyable experience for both handler and horse. As the animal gets into adolescence it will get cheeky, it will try to take advantage of you as it will have lost all fear of being in your company. Treat it like you would a spoiled child; DO NOT let it get away with any ill mannered behaviour. Raising the voice may be all that is required, but if it is not then a sharp slap as well as the voice will mostly suffice. While this is going on, you must have a firm grip of it with a leading rope attached to the headcollar, and do not let go! After you have sorted it out, then talk quietly and calmly again while clapping and stroking, to reassure that good behaviour is rewarded.

Vets as professional people do have to put themselves into potentially dangerous situations. While we can and do take as many precautions as we can to minimise the risks, it can only be asking for trouble to be standing at the rear end of a cow or horse with your arm stuck up one of its natural orifices.

I have a series of slides which I use to illustrate what I do when I am giving talks to Rotary or other such organisations. In one of these pictures I am viewed at the rear end of a patient with an expression on my face which was a mixture of concentration and fear. A member of one of my audiences told me that after seeing the Herriot films and now me "in action", he reckoned that all vets have an anal fixation. I was about to launch into a lengthy explanation about what I was doing and why, when I realised I was quietly having my leg pulled. I said instead, it was a cold day when the photograph was taken, and vets like everyone else liked to have a warm inside job when the weather was bad!

It's not only physical damage we might sustain in our dealings with animals. There are all manner of pests and diseases to which we can all prove susceptible. Some of these can be life threatening like Salmonellosis, or if you are abroad, Rabies. Others like ringworm or ticks or flea bites are usually just an irritation. If you are working with animals outdoors, particularly horses, then I make no apologies for emphasising the absolute necessity for being up to date with your anti tetanus vaccination. Horses and ponies are very prone to the ravages of this disease, and as the bacteria are commonly found in the soil, equines are often passing large quantities of the germ in their dung. All horses and donkeys should be regularly vaccinated, but so too should their handlers, as once the disease has a hold whether you are man or animal, the odds are very much against recovery. At least an animal, in extremes when there is no hope of recovery can be humanely put to sleep, but not so humans — yet.

RABIES

Rabies is a particularly horrifying disease which we can get from animals. The sight of a person dying from Rabies in convulsions and terrified of water, is very distressing. Perhaps the most terrifying part of it all is the knowledge that between convulsions, the person who is so afflicted is fully aware of what is going on. There is no cure once clinical symptoms have been established. This country, thanks to the effectiveness of the quarantine laws, has been free of the disease for many years. There is a strong movement afoot in the European Community with the advent of all frontier restrictions coming to an end, for Britain to relax its control and allow free passage of all animals within the Community.

Great improvements have been made on the continent in the control of the disease by using live vaccine in bait to inoculate the wildlife and foxes particularly. There is still much to be done before Rabies can be discounted as a threat, and we would be stupid to allow animals into the UK without restriction. If we did, we would be living under the constant threat of Rabies getting into the fox population of the country. All dogs would have to be registered whether the government liked it or not, and all dogs and cats would have to be inoculated against the disease, probably enforced by law.

FOOD POISONING

There are many different causes of food poisoning, most of which are the result of contamination of food by bacteria or the poisons from bacteria.

Salmonella infections in people is perhaps the most common cause of food poisoning and much has been made recently by the press discovery that eggs, not uncommonly carry the infection salmonella Enteritides. This fact has been known for many years by the veterinary profession and to a lesser extent by those in the poultry industry, but it came as a great shock to the British public. The sickness and diarrhoea that it can cause can be dangerous to the very young and the vulnerable old. However, many people were caused unnecessary worry due to all the journalistic hype, but some good came out of all the furore. Tighter hygiene controls were brought in, and swabs taken on a regular basis from all laying hens so that the risk to the public health from eggs was reduced to almost nothing.

RINGWORM

Ringworm, is one of three diseases where the name gives a totally wrong impression. It is a skin disease caused by fungus, not a worm. In horse, cattle and man it appears as a round raised lesion on the skin. Like this it is easy to diagnose, but in other animals like the dog, and in cats especially, it can require a laboratory test to confirm its presence.

The infection is very common in people who are handling cattle, and I am quite often asked to confirm an already suspected diagnosis. This can sometimes lead to marital strife, as in one occasion: I was asked my opinion as to what might be the cause of a red sore on a farmer's wife's abdomen. I said I thought it was due to ringworm and the lady was not very happy, as she immediately suspected the source of the infection was her husband's hand. She was probably right as she did not have any direct contact with the calves in the yard which had the infection. The treatment for people is for the Doctor to decide, but it does seem to take longer to cure a person than a cow. The prevention is to be as careful about personal hygiene as possible, and to treat all animals that have the disease.

Ringworm in your dog and cat is more difficult to diagnose as it is often caused by a different fungi to that in cattle and horses. The lesions will fluoresce under ultra violet light, turning a pale green colour which is a help in diagnosis. Cats often show very few signs of an infection, and it may not be suspected until a human has the classical signs and the household pet has to be screened. The treatment in cats can be a long drawn out affair. It is usually recommended that the drug Griseofulvin is given by mouth for up to three months at a time to be sure of a cure. This is in marked contrast to the treatment of horses and cattle, where the same treatment has only to be given for ten days for good results. Before griseofulvin was used to treat the disease, many cats had to be put down as they were a constant source of infection to others.

There is still a great deal of public ignorance and hysteria about the most talked about zoonosis, which is visceral larva migrans. This is the condition where children become infected with the immature stage of the dog roundworm, Toxocara Canis. The children most at risk are those who have close contact with household pets or who frequently use areas of public parks where there is contamination of the ground by dog faeces.

Surveys have shown that there is a high incidence of the worm eggs in soil samples, but despite this the reported incidence of clinical infection is very small. However, the cases that do occur can be serious as the larvae, once inside the child, can get into the circulation and find their way to the eye. This can, in some cases, result in blindness.

The treatment and control of the disease is simple, as the adult worm can easily be removed by most worming preparations. Puppies should be de-wormed from about two weeks of age and receive the medication every fortnight until they are three to four months old. Their mother should be treated at the same time until the puppies are weaned. Despite this blanket therapy, as there may be a few worms present even in adult dogs, I recommend that all adult dogs should be de-wormed twice a year. Despite the risk from cat round worms being very slight, it is still there, and I usually suggest that owners follow the same regime as for dogs.

Other control measures are based on common sense. Safe disposal of dog dirt is essential. Where your dog messes, clean it up, even if it is in your back garden, but particularly if you are in a public place. It's surprising, given the extent of public awareness about the risks of allowing your dog to eliminate in a public place, how casual a lot of breeders are about worming their own breeding bitches and puppies. They are not the only professionals who can be a bit unaware. A few months ago, a General Practitioner telephoned me about one of his patients. A little boy, about two years old, had eaten some dog faeces and he wondered what the risk was to the child. I thought the risk to the child was very small, but I did advise that the child be de-wormed at the appropriate time. The doctor had not given a thought to this at all, but at least he did take the trouble to find out.

Roundworms are not the only parasite that man can get from animals in this country. The adult tape worm, Taenia Saginata, which is found in people has its intermediate stage as a larve in the muscle tissue of cattle. My lecturer in parasitology at Vet School had just such an infection of which he seemed very proud. At least he tended to sign off his lectures with "Well that's about enough for now, I must go and feed Tommy." Tommy was the pet name for his beast. He assumed he had probably received the tape worm through his taste for eating his steak rare to almost raw, and he was paying for the consequences. It caused very little inconvenience apparently, except he tended to get hungry frequently, and his wife was not too pleased with the state of his underpants from time to time! The last was due to the tape worm segments having minds of their own, and coming out when least expected. He, at that time, had thought of trying to get rid of the pest, but the treatment was fairly drastic then, involving purgatives and other horrors. He decided, weighing everything in the balance, that the treatment might prove more hazardous to his system than living with Tommy. I occasionally wonder, now the medication is much more effective, whether he has bothered to get rid of the pest, but remembering his eccentricities, probably not! To be fair to the chap, he did warn us all most sternly against the risks of eating under cooked meat. He was especially concerned for the young ladies of the class in case any were tempted to get one for themselves, as it was a perfect way to eat as much as you liked and still stay nice and slim.

The detection of the parasite by modern methods of meat inspection has greatly reduced the odds of picking it up. Coupled with this, the practice of using human waste as a fertiliser on the fields where cattle graze has been discontinued, but I still prefer to have my steak well done!

Despite the potential hazards of internal parasites, the pest that seems to cause most revulsion in the consulting room is the flea, or worse still lice. The average client will recoil with disgust from a pet that has been demonstrated to be carrying a few extra "friends", and almost unconsciously start scratching. The treatments against external parasites have improved hugely since I qualified, but still the flea seems to be one jump ahead! Fleas are still the most common cause of itchiness and skin infections in dogs and cats. They seem to be more prevalent than ever. This is probably due, especially in the winter months, to many houses now having central heating. They love warm dark conditions to thrive and breed. Don't we all? Come the late spring or early summer there can be a sudden explosion in the numbers in a house, and the rooms can be quite literally crawling with the pests.

This happened to a friend's house. She only had a cat at the time, and despite being very house proud, she had to get the council in to fumigate her home. Fleas were swarming like bees from under the woodwork and all over the carpets. Her family had all come out in red itchy spots and refused to go home until something was done.

The family cat, the initial source of the infection, escaped with her life when I promised that a flea collar would prevent any reoccurrence of the infestation.

I often wonder what it is within our make up that causes many of us not to feel complete without having animals around, living and working with us. No doubt it goes back to our roots, when primeval man first shared a fire with a wild animal and was first aware how useful a trained beast could be. Certainly in my opinion, a house without a pet isn't a home, and a farm without animals is a barren, sterile place.

IT WAS CHRISTMAS TIME

It was Christmas time at the Practice,
And all the staff had gone home,
A thousand and one cases to deal with,
And here's me all on my own.

The above with apologies to Dickens and any poet that may be reading this, but it about sums up what Christmas has sometimes meant to me. I would not care for you to think it all bad, because it's not. It's like the curate egg; some are good, some are bad, and some are truly awful!

The pre-Christmas period is the same most years, normally hectic! Most farmers are very keen to get all the routine work out of the way before all the festivities start, as these days most farm workers tend to have one or two weeks of their holidays at this time. Small animal clients are often intent on getting their pets boostered before they are sent to the kennels for the duration of the break. This period of activity is made worse in the practice by everyone, not unnaturally, wanting the odd day off to get the final bits of last minute shopping. This leaves everyone else short tempered and irritable, having to cope with the extra work load. However, the busy run up to the holiday is brightened by the many cards we receive from grateful patients. We seldom get a card from an owner; there is always a remarkable outbreak of literacy by our canine, feline and occasionally equine patients. Somehow or other though, this doesn't ever seem to extend to cows, sheep or pigs; they never get to write. Perhaps the intensive farming in this area just doesn't give time for literary endeavours! We are also recipients of the occasional bottle of the stuff that cheers, and not a few boxes of mince pies! On two memorable Christmas Eve's in a row, one kind lady actually bought two cases (yes cases) of rather good wine for us all to share! Sadly she has now gone from the Fens. Our loss is Yorkshire's gain; as if that county hasn't got enough good things as it is!

The real start of Christmas for me is when the staff have gone home, the roads have quietened down, and it's only me, a few hospitalised patients, and my much put upon family. A good Christmas is one that has been so quiet that I am quite pleased to see a patient, even if it's the family dog almost choking on a stolen turkey bone. Memorable Christmases are, however, almost invariably hectic with particular cases long remembered.

Some years ago, I was called out at 8.30 in the evening to a cow having difficulty calving. She was in an old fashioned barn with some barely adequate light. She was a Friesian, in calf to a Charollais. Charollais is a continental breed of cattle, renowned for being large animals. British farmers use this and other foreign breeds crossed with the more traditional British breeds, to produce a larger calf which is worth a great deal more money. An examination of the patient didn't take long, and it was soon realised that due to the size of the calf, the only way to effect a safe delivery was by a Caesarian operation.

It's not a job lightly undertaken, as the operation as well as requiring the necessary surgical skills, needs at least two people who are reasonably strong and fit, as it is also a physically demanding procedure. My partner's help was forthcoming and together we set to work. The barn was quite warm, despite it being a cold night; the collective warmth of the other cattle, coupled with the heat from the extra light which we had rigged up to enable us to see what we were doing, even had us sweating a bit.

An incision was made in the cow's left side about twenty minutes after the local anaesthetic was given. The many muscle layers were divided to enable us to penetrate the abdominal wall and locate the uterus. Due to the size of the calf, it was impossible to bring the womb out to the surface of the skin layers. This is the normal procedure to enable an accurate incision into the uterus. This time I had to take the scalpel into the abdomen and do the job blind, by touch only.

With this accomplished, the next move was to pull the calf out. We couldn't do it! It was so large and heavy that even with out collective strengths we just could not lift it out through the open wound. Fortunately, with great presence of mind, the farmer quickly got a block and tackle attached to the roof beams, and with ropes tied to the front feet of the calf, it was soon lifted up and out. It was a bull calf, and he was enormous!

As in the best fishing stories where the weight of the fish gets exaggerated with the passing of the years, so it is with the birth weights of calves, but this one must have been over two hundred pounds.

By good fortune he was alive, and the mother who seemed very unimpressed by the whole affair, was eventually and with some difficulty, put back together again. Whilst we were stitching her up, the farmer went off, he said for some more clean water, and came back from the house with a bottle of whisky. We drank a toast in the best tradition, to Christmas and to the new born infant.

Which brings me to one of the more trying aspects of the festive season. Where ever you go, be it on Christmas Eve, Christmas Day or Boxing Day, there seems to be a party going on, to which you are often invited to join and partake in a little of the festive cheer. These days with everyone so aware of the perils of drinking and driving, this cheer has to be confined to consuming the odd mince pie or Christmas cake with a cup of coffee. It wasn't always like that, as I can remember all too well. Christmas is always associated in most people's minds with shepherds and lambs, and so it is with me. One of the best friends I have ever made I got to know very well one Christmas night.

He was a sheep farmer, and called me to a ewe having difficulties lambing. It was about 2am, the night was bright and clear, being a time of a full moon, with more than a touch of frost in the air.

The mother to be was in a pen in the lambing yard, and I attended to her with a brisk efficiency and considering it was the middle of the night, commendable good humour. The ewe had a minor presentation problem with her lambs in that both wanted to be born at the same time. It was merely a matter of pushing one back and sorting out which legs belonged to which lamb. Once this was accomplished, the ewe almost managed the rest for herself.

As I was packing up my gear afterwards in the barn, I couldn't help noticing that Mike, the farmer, had a bottle of malt whisky in the feed bin. Out of somewhere he conjured up two fairly clean glasses, and I sat on a feed bag and gave my considered opinion as to the quality of his whisky. it was a serious matter which took some time and a lot of discussion, and we adjourned to the house to consider our musings in greater comfort. Two hours passed as if in a moment, and I suddenly realised to my horror that it was almost 4am and I hadn't left a note as to where I was or what I was doing! I rushed off home hoping that there hadn't been another call and my wife wasn't waiting up worrying about where I was and whether I had had an accident.

I needn't have worried, as when I reached home smelling like a distillery, she was still sound asleep and blissfully unaware of my nocturnal misdemeanours. I made a ewe comfortable, saved two lambs lives, and made a life long friend that night, but it's not a procedure I would dare to repeat today. Except I do still enjoy his whisky, I now just don't drive afterwards!

Patients that refuse to get better despite all the best of modern medicine, are a pain at the best of time, but when it happens on Christmas Day itself, they can be very trying indeed. Colic is an affliction which can happen at any time, but always seems to have a timing all of its own. A common cause of colic, or stomach pain in the horse is constipation, and as previously mentioned, is usually the result of eating something unsuitable like the straw bedding.

This particular mare became quite ill early on Christmas Day morning. On attending it was obvious that the animal was very bunged up, and was given as well as a pain killer, a very large dose (about a gallon) of liquid paraffin by stomach tube. She was revisited four more times that day, a round trip of some twenty miles. Each time she had to have more pain killing injections as well as more fluids as she slowly, oh so slowly, got rid of her burden.

Boxing Day arrived to find that the mare had finally succeeded in clearing herself, and there was a satisfying pile of dung in the corner of the stable, and a further mess halfway up the wall! She had a smile on her face almost as big as my own, as I was beginning to think that only a stick of dynamite would do the job!

Sad moments occur all too often as well. Another calving I will never forget happened about six years ago on a Boxing Day night. The patient was a little heifer with a very large dead calf inside her. It was a night of freezing fog, and chilling certainty that to relieve her of her calf would take many hours of hard labour. The only way to save the beast, as the calf had been dead for a good few hours, was to dismember it while it was still inside her and remove it in pieces. A Caesarean operation at this stage, due to the sepsis in the womb, would mean almost certain death to the heifer. It is almost impossible during a Caesarean operation to stop the contents of the uterus leaking into the abdomen. If the calf has been dead for any length of time, and operation would result in peritonitis and death of the patient.

The alternative to the Caesarean, the embryotomy procedure, is conducted though the vagina. Various instruments, including cutting wire like robust cheese wire, are used to remove the limbs and the other parts from the body, until all can be removed with the minimum amount of stress to the mother. It's a difficult, tiring, messy job at the best of times, but that night, in that weather realising the trauma the heifer was going through, everyone's Christmas spirit was at an all time low. The operation took from about nine pm until nearly one am, and I have rarely felt so tired and fed up after a job. The heifer survived the experience, but only just, and was never fit to breed again.

I have had well over twenty Christmases in the Practice, and in many ways they have all seemed very similar, except that my children have got older and now moved away from home. Last year, for the first time since I became a vet, I spent Christmas away from the practice, back in my native Scotland. I can say I had a memorable time, but I also must be honest and confess there were times when I half missed the strident tones of the summoning telephone to another emergency. If nothing else, it used to get me out of doing the washing up!

Also published by Smallholder Publications Ltd

SMALLHOLDER Magazine
The practical monthly for the small farmer

and the

SMALLHOLDER PRACTICAL SERIES

Introduction to Goat Keeping
by Jenny Neal

Smallholders and Farmers Legal Handbook
by John Clarke

Plain and Simple Egg Production
by Carol Twinch

So You Want to Keep Seep
by Carol Twinch

Successful Lambing for the Small Flock Owner
by John Bartelous

Pig Rearing and Health
by R. Russell Lyon

A Guide to Angora-Cross Goats for Meat & Fibre
by Joanna and David Charman